ESSENTIALS About
the **GYNAECOLOGIC EXAM**

R. Mimi Secor, DNP, FNP-BC, FAANP, is a nurse practitioner (NP), national speaker/educator, and consultant. She has worked for 40 years as a family nurse practitioner specializing in women's health. In 2015, she earned her doctor of nursing practice degree from Rocky Mountain University of Health Professions in Provo, Utah. Dr. Secor is a guest lecturer at NP programs in New England and around the country. She has published extensively; her 2014 coauthored textbook, *Advanced Health Assessment of Women: Skills and Procedures,* was selected as a 2015 American Journal of Nursing award winner. In 2012, Dr. Secor coauthored the first edition of the Essentials title *Essentials About the Gynaecologic Exam for Nurse Practitioners: Conducting the GYN Exam in a Nutshell.* Dr. Secor has received several awards, including the 2013 Lifetime Achievement Award from the Massachusetts Coalition of Nurse Practitioners, and the 2015 Student Service Award from Rocky Mountain University for her contributions to the NP profession.

Heidi Collins Fantasia, PhD, RN, WHNP-BC, is an associate professor at Zuckerberg College of Health Sciences, Susan and Alan Solomont School of Nursing, at the University of Massachusetts, Lowell, and a visiting scholar at the William F. Connell School of Nursing at Boston College. Dr. Fantasia is a women's health nurse practitioner who provides contraceptive and reproductive health care for a Title X family-planning clinic in northeastern Massachusetts. She has more than 25 years of clinical nursing experience, including inpatient obstetrics and advanced practice women's health care in both private and public health settings. Dr. Fantasia has authored more than 50 peer-reviewed publications on a variety of topics related to women's health and has presented her work nationally and internationally. She conducts research in the area of reproductive health with a specific focus on the intersection of physical and sexual violence and women's reproductive health.

ESSENTIALS About the **GYNAECOLOGIC EXAM**

A Professional Guide for NPs, PAs, and Midwives

Second Edition

R. Mimi Secor, DNP, FNP-BC, FAANP
Heidi Collins Fantasia, PhD, RN, WHNP-BC

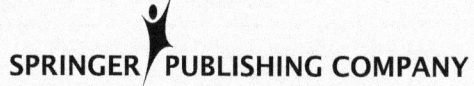

Copyright © 2018 Springer Publishing Company, LLC

All rights reserved.

No part of this publication may be reproduced, stored in a retrieval system, or transmitted in any form or by any means, electronic, mechanical, photocopying, recording, or otherwise, without the prior permission of Springer Publishing Company, LLC, or authorization through payment of the appropriate fees to the Copyright Clearance Center, Inc., 222 Rosewood Drive, Danvers, MA 01923, 978-750-8400, fax 978-646-8600, or on the Web at www.copyright.com.

Springer Publishing Company, LLC
11 West 42nd Street
New York, NY 10036
www.springerpub.com

Acquisitions Editor: Elizabeth Nieginski
Senior Production Editor: Kris Parrish
Compositor: Westchester Publishing Services

ISBN: 978-0-8261-3473-8

The author and the publisher of this Work have made every effort to use sources believed to be reliable to provide information that is accurate and compatible with the standards generally accepted at the time of publication. Because medical science is continually advancing, our knowledge base continues to expand. Therefore, as new information becomes available, changes in procedures become necessary. We recommend that the reader always consult current research and specific institutional policies before performing any clinical procedure. The author and publisher shall not be liable for any special, consequential, or exemplary damages resulting, in whole or in part, from the readers' use of, or reliance on, the information contained in this book. The publisher has no responsibility for the persistence or accuracy of URLs for external or third-party Internet websites referred to in this publication and does not guarantee that any content on such websites is, or will remain, accurate or appropriate.

> Contact us to receive discount rates on bulk purchases.
> We can also customize our books to meet your needs.
> For more information please contact: sales@springerpub.com

The ESSENTIALS series was published in the United States by Springer Publishing Company, LLC, as the FAST FACTS series.

Contents

Contributor — ix
Foreword   Joellen W. Hawkins, PhD, RN, WHNP-BC — xi
Preface — xiii
Acknowledgments — xv

Part I   INTRODUCTION TO THE GYNAECOLOGIC EXAM

1. **Conducting the Interview and Taking a Gynaecologic and Sexual History** — 3
   R. Mimi Secor

2. **The Abdominal Exam** — 15
   R. Mimi Secor

3. **The Vulvar Exam** — 21
   R. Mimi Secor

4. **The Speculum Exam** — 37
   R. Mimi Secor

5. **The Bimanual Exam** — 53
   R. Mimi Secor

6. **The Rectal Exam** — 61
   R. Mimi Secor

Part II   APPROACH TO EXAMINING SPECIAL POPULATIONS

7. **Specific "Challenges"** — 71
   Heidi Collins Fantasia

8. **Examining the Woman With Anxiety, History of Sexual Violence, or Intimate Partner Violence**   79
Heidi Collins Fantasia

9. **Examining Premenarchal Children, Adolescents, and Virginal Women**   93
Heidi Collins Fantasia

10. **Useful Techniques When Examining Overweight, Multiparous, or Physically Challenged Women**   101
Heidi Collins Fantasia

11. **Special Considerations When Examining the Postmenopausal and Older Woman**   111
Heidi Collins Fantasia

12. **Care of the Woman Who Has Experienced Female Genital Mutilation**   121
Heidi Collins Fantasia

13. **Gynaecological Examination of the Transgender Patient**   129
Teri Bunker

Appendices   *137*
   A. Common Pelvic Examination Problems and Interventions   *139*
   B. Vaginal Microscopy Flow Sheet   *141*
   C. Vaginal Microscopy: Flow Sheet Instructions   *143*
   D. Vulvar Care Guidelines for Patient Education   *145*
Bibliography   *147*
Abbreviations   *151*
Index   *155*

Contributor

Teri Bunker, DNP, FNP
Family Nurse Practitioner
Bridge City Family Medical Clinic
Portland, Oregon

Foreword

This new edition is an extraordinarily down-to-earth and useful guide for both novice clinicians and experienced clinicians who are presented with challenging patient situations. The format facilitates both a rapid review immediately prior to stepping into the examination room, as well as a more leisurely study in anticipation of a new clinical challenge, or a prospective roster of patients.

The authors have both synthesized and explained the most important aspects of, preparation for, and conduction of a gynaecologic examination under what are sometimes less-than-ideal circumstances. Their writing is succinct, clear, and easy to read and meets their goal of providing guidance for novice clinicians, as well as providing a quick review for experienced clinicians about to examine patients with unusual or unfamiliar characteristics.

Most of all, this book is a gold mine for clinicians committed to delivering the best possible care to women who present with a wide range of characteristics and challenges. Equally so, it should become a must-have book for novice clinicians as they struggle to make it through their first solo gynaecologic examination, and move on to mastering the art of caregiving as well as the science of providing the best possible individualized care for each woman across the life span.

Joellen W. Hawkins, PhD, RN, WHNP-BC
Professor Emeritus, William F. Connell School of Nursing, Boston College
Chestnut Hill, Massachusetts

Preface

Many advanced practice clinicians (nurse practitioners [NPs], physician assistants [PAs], certified nurse-midwives [CNMs]) lack confidence in their women's health skills and may be particularly apprehensive and unsure of their gynaecologic exam skills. We have written this book because there is a great need for practical information about how to improve the advanced practice clinician's gynaecologic exam skills.

Essentials About the Gynaecologic Exam represents the coauthors' more than four decades of combined clinical experience in women's health and teaching NPs and other advanced practice clinicians how to perform gynaecologic examinations.

This practical guide is designed in an easy-to-follow format well suited for the busy clinician looking to refine his or her skills, or for students just learning how to perform a gynaecologic exam and the instructors/preceptors who are assisting them.

Each chapter in this book contains key learning objectives and content related to the specific aspect of the gynaecologic exam being discussed. We have included detailed suggestions, approaches, and step-by-step sequences on how to perform the various aspects of the gynaecologic exam. Tapping into our vast combined clinical experiences, we have included many practical suggestions both in the body of the text and in the "Essential Facts" sections of each chapter. These special Essentials sections contain clinical pearls intended to help clinicians improve their skills so they can conduct a better exam.

There are also helpful figures to illustrate information and procedures being discussed.

The text and appendices provide valuable guidelines and documents, including suggestions and strategies for various gynaecologic exam challenges and dealing with special populations, a vaginal microscopy flow sheet and summary of how to perform this test and document your results, the new cervical cancer screening guidelines, how to perform an anal Papanicolau smear, and patient education guidelines for vulvovaginal self-care.

This book will help advanced practice clinicians develop and refine their gynaecologic examination skills so they can perform a more accurate, patient-centered exam with confidence. This new edition will be a welcome resource, especially for students and their instructors.

R. Mimi Secor
Heidi Collins Fantasia

Acknowledgments

Thanks to my coauthor, Dr. Heidi Fantasia, who is a great writer and with whom it was a pleasure to work on this second edition. I am indebted to the patients I have encountered over the years. They are a source of inspiration as I continually learn so much from them. Thank you to the friends, students, and nurse practitioner colleagues for their insight, inspiration, support, and friendship. Special thanks to Dr. Joellen Hawkins, for being a dear friend and a career-long mentor, and to Teri Bunker, for writing our new chapter on care of the transgender patient. Finally, thanks to my family, including my husband, Mike, daughter, Katherine, and mother, Irene Clarke, for their unconditional love and for sharing me with my work.

R. Mimi Secor

Thank you to Mimi Secor for the wonderful opportunity to contribute to this project. I am forever grateful to my patients, colleagues, and coworkers, who have provided valuable stories, shared life experiences, and taught me to challenge myself and never stop learning. I would especially like to acknowledge Dr. Joellen Hawkins for being a longtime mentor and friend. I appreciate the unconditional love, support, and strength from my family, including my mother, Gretchen Collins, my husband, John, and my children, Andrew, Amelia, and Evan.

Heidi Collins Fantasia

Introduction to the Gynaecologic Exam

Conducting a gynaecologic exam requires many clinical skills. These include competence in establishing and building emotional rapport with women; knowing how and what questions to ask to elicit an appropriate gynaecologic history; conducting a systematic, thorough, and accurate pelvic exam in a confident, reassuring manner; and documenting medical records appropriately. Frequently, this involves the use of electronic medical records, including transmitting prescriptions electronically.

1

Conducting the Interview and Taking a Gynaecologic and Sexual History

R. Mimi Secor

The gynaecologic exam visit involves many competencies, skills, and steps, including taking a gynaecologic history, conducting a gynaecologic exam, using excellent communication and clinical skills, and the ability to formulate a management plan to address preventive goals and health issues pertinent to the individual woman. This process is complex and individualized to each woman and situation. Knowledge, practice, and experience are required to develop basic competency and, with time, expert skills.

In this chapter, you will learn how to:

- Develop skills and strategies for creating a therapeutic environment for conducting a gynaecologic exam
- Obtain key elements of a gynaecologic history
- Take a gynaecologic history, including how to ask questions particularly related to taking a sexual history

CREATING A THERAPEUTIC ENVIRONMENT

The environment that welcomes the woman into the office setting establishes the stage. There are many elements to take into consideration when designing and furnishing a waiting room or area. For example, introducing "comfort" measures into the waiting area communicates that the woman is expected and welcomed. These measures can include comfortable chairs; current magazines; pleasant art on the walls; and access to a water cooler with disposable cups, which can each contribute to increasing her feeling of being welcomed and comfortable upon arrival. Train the reception personnel to be pleasant, to call the woman by name, to provide easy instructions for completing needed paperwork, and to offer directions to the bathroom, all of which can contribute to helping her relax.

PRE-APPOINTMENT INSTRUCTIONS

Before the appointment, the woman should be advised to avoid intravaginal medications, douching, and intercourse within 24 hours of her visit. This improves diagnostic accuracy by minimizing disruptions in the vaginal ecosystem potentially caused by these factors.

ESTABLISHING RAPPORT

It is important to establish and maintain effective rapport with the woman and to incorporate various approaches to facilitate this process. This begins when the clinician introduces herself or himself to each patient, giving his or her full name and professional title of nurse practitioner.

ESSENTIAL FACTS

One should always shake the woman's hand (perhaps not during flu season). This establishes physical contact, respect, friendliness, and equality. This is the first opportunity for body contact (a gradual approach is good) and is an important component of the gynaecologic examination.

Other strategies to help establish rapport include the following:

Professional Image

The clinician should dress professionally and wear a name tag in a visible location on his or her lab coat, scrubs, or clothing. Some clinicians opt not to wear a lab coat; if they choose to wear street clothes, these should be appropriate to the clinician's setting, community, and patient population (always clean and wrinkle free) and communicate a professional image.

The Initial Conversation

Help the woman feel comfortable by asking about her occupation and family and how her day is going. At first glance this may seem like small talk, but it provides an opportunity to establish a rapport before transitioning into the reason for her visit. This initial conversation helps establish rapport, breaks the ice, and sets the tone for the visit and relationship.

Communicate About the Role of the Nurse Practitioner

Ask the patient whether she has seen a nurse practitioner before; this can create an opportunity to educate about nurse practitioners, including discussion about the clinician's particular specialty, her or his position in the practice, experience, and expertise. The clinician might want to discuss how the woman can address the clinician, for example, Dr. Secor or Mimi. The clinician can also ask, particularly if she is older than the patient, how the patient would like to be addressed, by first name or by marital status and last name.

Use Humor

Use appropriate humor to help the woman relax. For example, saying something like, "Men don't know what courage is; it's making a gyn exam appointment and keeping it!" This helps create a moment of levity and bonding. Do, however, avoid inappropriate humor.

INTRODUCTION TO DOCUMENTING THE GYNAECOLOGIC EXAM

The Electronic Medical Record

The advantages of using an electronic medical record (EMR) include enhanced accuracy of documentation and greater opportunity for women to participate in and negotiate the specific data that are recorded (medicolegal implications). Also, when the clinician becomes proficient, EMR use can actually improve efficiency.

When using EMRs during the interview, the clinician should position the computer to facilitate optimal eye contact and promote ergonomic comfort for both the woman and examiner. The clinician should inform the woman that it may be necessary to periodically interrupt the conversation to accurately record findings during the visit. This requires a certain level of proficiency; otherwise, she may feel that the clinician is not fully listening to her. Predesigned EMR templates facilitate communication, provide a systematic structure for the workup, ensure inclusion of the key elements of the assessment, and potentially save time.

Examples of documenting a gynaecologic exam visit are provided in sections throughout the next few chapters, as the gynaecologic exam is described.

ESSENTIAL FACTS

Documenting as you progress through the patient visit increases accuracy of data reporting and improves proficiency of EMR use.

INTRODUCTION TO CONDUCTING THE MEDICAL INTERVIEW

Conduct the initial interview in a private location, with the woman fully clothed, and with both the examiner and the woman sitting in relatively close proximity. Inform her that the conversation and care are confidential per the Health Insurance Portability and Accountability Act (HIPAA) of 1996 and that questions the clinician asks her are to help provide the highest quality individualized care, including diagnosis and management of the woman's problems. Note the general appearance of the woman as the clinician conducts the interview and prepares to examine the patient.

Obtain the General Medical History

It is important to elicit a general medical history, being careful to include the following elements:

- Current medical history, including review of systems (ROS)
- Past medical and surgical history
- Family history
- Allergies to medications
- Medications, including nonprescription and over-the-counter medications taken; herbs; homeopathics; and supplements
- Health maintenance, such as last Papanicolaou (Pap) smear, mammogram, colonoscopy, bone density test, and so forth
- Vaccination status
- Social history
  - Occupation, work, home, family, friend network, spiritual base, leisure activities
  - Smoking, alcohol use, recreational drug use
  - Exercise, sleep, stress, diet, nutritional status
  - Abuse history
  - Safe-sex practices
  - Distracted driving, seat belts

Obtain the Gynaecologic History

The clinician should begin obtaining the gynaecologic history by asking about related problems and taking a detailed history of these problems.

The menstrual history includes the following elements:

- Age of menarche
- Cycle interval (approximately 28 days)
- Duration and amount of flow
- Date (first day) of last menstrual period (LMP)
- Associated menstrual symptoms
  - Recent changes in menses
  - Premenstrual symptoms

- Menorrhagia
- Dysmenorrhea (onset, duration, self-management)
- Late or lighter menses (suspected pregnancy) and associated pregnancy symptoms
- History of unprotected intercourse since LMP (must rule out pregnancy)

ESSENTIAL FACTS

If the woman reports unprotected intercourse, inconsistent use of birth control, or a later, lighter menses, you must rule out pregnancy. This is especially important if she is complaining of pregnancy symptoms, such as breast tenderness, urinary frequency, fatigue, and/or nausea.

Ask the woman about menstrual history since menarche, being careful to obtain details about the occurrence of:

- Amenorrhea
- Oligomenorrhea
- Pregnancy
- Irregular or abnormal uterine bleeding (AUB), formerly known as dysfunctional uterine bleeding (DUB)
- Spotting

ESSENTIAL FACTS

- A history of irregular menses since menarche, especially if there is significant irregularity (skipping months numerous times over 1 or more years), should prompt the clinician to consider the diagnosis of polycystic ovarian syndrome (PCOS).
- Significant dysmenorrhea and dyspareunia over months and/or years may suggest endometriosis or pelvic inflammatory disease (PID).

Obtain Sexual History

Sexual history is a key component of a gynaecologic history. How the clinician asks questions and creates an environment conducive to disclosure are both critically important factors in taking a sexual history. A clinician must help women feel comfortable discussing their sexuality. Also, the clinician needs to take care in avoiding a heterosexual bias.

- Ask about past and current sexual activity.
- Note age of first intercourse, also referred to as *coitarche*.
- Estimate the total number of sexual partners the woman has been involved with (including genders and estimated percentage of time condoms used with intercourse). This information helps the clinician to evaluate the woman's risk for pregnancy, cervical cancer, and other sexually transmitted infections (STIs).
- If the woman is currently sexually active, ask whether her partner is male or female, whether she has more than one partner, and whether the woman and/or her partners are having sex with men, women, or both.
- Note the duration of her current relationship, along with the date of last intercourse, or sexual relations.
- Ask whether the relationship is monogamous; this is critical, as this information helps the examiner assess STI risk and the need for STI testing.
- Even though the woman may not currently have a sexual partner, she may still be sexually active; ask about utilization of sex toys or other forms of self-stimulation, including masturbation.
- Ask about specific sexual practices, including a history of penile/vaginal intercourse, oral/genital receptive sex, and/or anal receptive intercourse.
- Ask about condom use and estimate the percentage of times condoms were used; both are critical to assessing STI and pregnancy risk.
- Elicit and note past or current history of STIs, including both the type and dates of infections, treatment (if known), and any complications or sequelae such as chronic pelvic pain or infertility.

- Ascertain the date when the woman was last tested for STIs, including specific tests and the results. If the woman has current symptoms of a possible STI or vaginitis, elicit a history of present illness, including chief complaint, symptoms, and associated symptoms.

Pap Smear History

Obtain the woman's Pap smear history, as this is critical when evaluating current and past Pap smear results and is important when determining appropriate frequency of screening intervals.

- Ask for date of most recent Pap smear and the results.
- Obtain patient report of abnormal Pap smears in the past, including the dates, any follow-up such as colposcopy and biopsies, and follow-up Pap results.
- Follow the new cervical cancer screening guidelines that recommend the first Pap smear test be conducted at age 21, every 3 years until age 30, then every 5 years when combined with hr-HPV testing. (NOTE: hr-HPV is high risk subtypes of HPV).
- Advise women that they may consider discontinuing Pap screenings after age 65 if low risk (i.e., negative screening in the past 10 years and no history of cervical intraepithelial neoplasia [CIN] 2, 3).

History of Urinary Tract Infections

Elicit a history of urinary tract infections (UTIs), including current symptoms, past infections, total number of infections, history of genitourinary surgery or diagnostic tests such as cystoscopy, or urodynamic testing. Asking about a history of urinary tract symptoms or UTIs is an important part of the gynaecologic history because these problems may be associated with gynaecologic conditions such as vaginitis or STIs such as genital herpes. UTIs may also be caused by or aggravated by intercourse and/or atrophic vaginitis.

Contraceptive History

Taking a comprehensive contraceptive history is also a key component of the gynaecologic history. Include questions about:

- Her current contraceptive method, if any
- Level of satisfaction with the method
- Compliance with the method
- Side effects experienced
- Elicit questions/concerns about current method
- Past methods used and level of satisfaction or problems associated with these methods
- Unplanned pregnancies, complications, side effects, and other concerns

ESSENTIAL FACTS

A personal or family history, especially of cardiovascular problems, stroke, migraines with aura, or coagulopathies, is important to elicit, especially if the woman is considering combination hormonal contraceptives.

ASSESS VITAL SIGNS

Assess specific vital signs based on the reason for the visit and the nature of her complaint and clinical problem. If she has presented for a well-woman exam, it is reasonable and appropriate to assess full vital signs, including blood pressure, heart rate, weight, body mass index, and height. If she has presented for a problem, such as vaginitis, it may not be necessary or appropriate to assess full vital signs. However, whenever she complains of fever, significant abdominal pain, malaise, or urinary tract symptoms, it is appropriate and essential to assess temperature, blood pressure, and heart rate as well. During this part of the interview, the clinician will begin to determine exam components that should be performed based on the woman's vital signs.

Weight

Assess her weight during a well-woman visit and when indicated based on history. If the clinician notes or the woman reports a significant change, assessing weight is even more important. During any visit, women may ask to have their weight checked regardless of the type of visit.

Vital Signs

- Assess blood pressure when the woman reports any or all of the following symptoms:
  - Significant abdominal pain
  - Abnormal vaginal bleeding
  - Dizziness
  - Weakness

Promptly assess her blood pressure if PID, tubal pregnancy, or abnormal vaginal bleeding are suspected, or if the woman appears pale, weak, disoriented, diaphoretic, septic, or very ill or in significant pain. Include assessment of heart rate and respiratory rate in each of the following clinical situations.

- Assess heart and respiratory rates:
  - As part of a well-woman exam
  - During problem visits as indicated
  - If the woman appears ill or has constitutional symptoms, or the examiner suspects a significant infection
  - If the woman reports heart or respiratory problems or complaints
- Assess the woman's temperature in any of the following clinical situations:
  - Urinary tract symptoms
  - Abdominal pain, especially lower or flank areas
  - Pain with intercourse
  - Vaginal discharge or vaginitis complaints
  - Abnormal vaginal bleeding, irregular or heavy menses

ESSENTIAL FACTS

Assess her temperature after the gynaecologic exam, especially if you suspect PID even with only mild tenderness on examination of the uterus and/or adnexal area.

Performing additional nongynaecologic examination components is determined by the purpose of the visit, the woman's complaints or problems, and findings from other aspects of the physical exam performed thus far.

TRANSITIONING TO CONDUCTING THE GYNAECOLOGIC EXAM

On completion of the interview and obtaining her gynaecologic and sexual history, the clinician will begin to transition to the actual gynaecologic exam. Ask the woman to empty her bladder before the examination and collect a urine sample for testing, if indicated. Testing may include a urine dipstick screen, urinalysis, culture, pregnancy test, and STI testing.

In general, conduct the nongynaecologic aspects of the physical exam before the gynaecologic exam. This helps the woman become comfortable with the clinician. When conducting the physical examination, we recommend a head-to-toe sequence. There may be exceptions in which the clinician and/or the woman prefers to proceed to the gynaecologic exam, such as a history of vulvovaginitis, extreme anxiety, sexual abuse, patient requests, or other specific considerations. These special situations have been discussed in more detail in Part II.

2

The Abdominal Exam

R. Mimi Secor

Performing a thorough abdominal exam is recommended as part of most gynaecologic exams, regardless of the complaint or reason for the visit, and is included as part of a well-woman exam. Findings derived from this exam provide valuable information to assist in making an appropriate diagnostic assessment. Both reassuringly normal and abnormal clinical findings of concern can be elicited from performing a thorough abdominal exam. These may include changes in bowel sounds, tenderness (especially rebound), and palpable masses.

In this chapter, you will learn:

- The indications for performing an abdominal exam focusing on urogynaecologic complaints
- The technique and sequence for performing the abdominal exam
- Normal versus abnormal exam findings (Table 2.1)

The abdominal examination should precede the gynaecologic examination, as it provides clues to the nature of the complaint and may also reduce anxiety associated with anticipating the gynaecologic examination. This may not be the case if the woman has a history of sexual abuse (see Chapter 8).

Table 2.1

Assessment Findings of the Abdomen: Normal and Abnormal

Findings of area assessed

Normal	Abnormal
Contour and shape are symmetrical, no distention, peristalsis is present	Distention may indicate fibroid tumor, pregnancy, or other masses
Umbilicus is normal location and skin color	Periumbilical ecchymosis (Cullen's sign) is a classic sign of ruptured ectopic pregnancy
	Spider angiomas, commonly associated with pregnancy, appear just above the umbilicus between the second and fifth months
Skin is blemish free and may be lightly covered with hair	Rashes; lesions, such as PUPP, appear as coalescing papules on the abdomen (rarely near the umbilicus) during the last trimester and resolve postpartum; burns may indicate abuse; scars should be investigated related to past surgeries, including hysterectomies
Diastasis recti muscle should be smooth and firm	Separation of the abdominal rectus muscles (results of pregnancy, multiparity, congenital weakness, marked obesity)
Presence of striae (linea alba) is common from skin stretched during pregnancy	Purple lines may suggest Cushing's disease
Palpation of lower abdomen is normally nontender and pain free	Tenderness in presence of reported pelvic pain suggests PID, ectopic pregnancy, ovarian cyst, or urinary tract infection. Tenderness may also suggest appendicitis, especially if in right lower quadrant
Inguinal lymph nodes are soft, mobile, and nontender	Enlarged, soft, and tender nodes indicate STIs such as herpes simplex virus Hard, irregular, immobile nodes require referral to a specialist

(continued)

Table 2.1

Assessment Findings of the Abdomen: Normal and Abnormal (*continued*)

Findings of area assessed

Normal	Abnormal
Bowel sounds	Absence of bowel sounds may suggest acute abdomen, obstruction, ruptured appendicitis, and so forth
	Increased bowel sounds may be present with PID, gastrointestinal infections/conditions, and sepsis

PID, pelvic inflammatory disease; PUPP, pruritic urticarial papules of pregnancy; STIs, sexually transmitted infections.

Source: Adapted from Carcio and Secor (2015); Rhoads (2006).

Indications for a gynaecologic exam focusing on urogynaecologic complaints include:

- Constitutional symptoms: fever, chills, malaise, nausea, vomiting
- Urinary tract symptoms
- Abdominal pain, especially in lower or flank areas
- Dyspareunia (pain with intercourse)
- Vaginal discharge
- Abnormal vaginal bleeding, irregular or heavy menses
- Missed, late menses
- Follow-up exam as indicated, especially if you suspect pelvic inflammatory disease (PID), even with mild tenderness on examination of the uterus and adnexae

Gloves are optional during the abdominal exam unless the woman has open or moist lesions or if the lower abdominal exam involves assessing the upper genital area. This includes the groin, mons, and suprapubic areas.

Position the woman in a supine or low semi-Fowler's position while standing to her right side. This is not always possible depending on the layout of the examination room. Throughout the exam, closely monitor the woman's facial expressions for signs of discomfort and evidence of anxiety. This is particularly important when assessing severity of pain or tenderness reported during the history.

If the woman is in severe discomfort (even at rest), she is likely to be unable to lie on the exam table in a fully supine position with her legs extended flat on the exam table. She may prefer to bend her knees and may not be able to lie still or concentrate on the conversation or examination. Note whether she appears to be in mild, moderate, or severe distress. Also, observe whether she appears pale, apprehensive, diaphoretic, weak, withdrawn, restless, or uncooperative.

It is recommended that clinicians wash their hands in front of the woman just prior to commencing the exam. This practice serves both to consistently maintain a clean environment and to reassure the woman. Researchers have demonstrated that women feel more confident with clinicians who wash their hands in front of them.

ESSENTIAL FACTS

If the woman is ticklish, it may be helpful to start the examination by placing the woman's hand under or on top of the clinician's hand.

If the woman complains of urinary tract symptoms, it is important to assess for pyelonephritis by checking for costovertebral angle tenderness (CVAT), particularly if associated constitutional symptoms, such as fever, chills, weakness, nausea, or vomiting, are noted.

To assess for CVAT, stand behind the woman, placing the palm of one hand over the lateral aspect of the woman's midthoracic area. With the fist of the other hand, gently hit the top of the hand placed on the woman's back. If this maneuver causes discomfort in the woman, the test is considered positive for CVAT, indicating possible pyelonephritis.

If the woman is complaining of abdominal pain, it is essential to perform a thorough abdominal exam. The order of the abdominal exam is as follows (Exhibit 2.1):

1. Observation/inspection
2. Auscultation for bowel sounds

Exhibit 2.1

Procedure for Performing the Abdominal Exam

- Observe/inspect: Begin the abdominal exam with observation.
    - Inspect for asymmetry and abdominal distention.
    - Note any scars that may include surgical or abuse scars, rashes, or lesions.
    - Observe for Cullen's sign (ecchymosis around the umbilicus, ruptured ectopic pregnancy, or intraperitoneal bleeding).
    - Observe for Grey Turner's sign (ecchymosis in flank area)—may indicate previous abdominal trauma or abuse.
- Next, auscultate the abdomen for bowel sounds in all four quadrants.
    - Note sounds as normal, absent, abnormally loud bowel sounds (referred to as *borborygmi*).
    - Sounds may be high pitched (normal small intestine) or low pitched and rumbling (large intestine).
    - Lack of bowel sounds may suggest an obstruction, whereas abnormally loud bowel sounds—borborygmi—may indicate some other type of gastrointestinal problem.
- Percuss the abdomen by placing your middle finger on the abdomen and tapping over the tip of that finger with the middle finger of the other hand.
    - High-pitched sounds might suggest a distended abdomen.
    - Dull sounds might suggest enlarged organs or mass(es).
    - Palpate, first lightly using the palm of your hand, then deeper using palmer surfaces of extended fingers, applying firm pressure with second hand on top to deliver deeper pressure. Include assessment of possible rebound tenderness.
    - Goal of light palpation is to assess areas of reported pain or tenderness.
    - Examine the quadrant in which pain has been reported last, to avoid tensing of muscles.
    - *Rebound tenderness* is defined as the woman describing more pain upon release of the palpation.
    - Note essentials caution.
- For complaints of lower abdominal pain or unusual tenderness in a woman, it is important to consider a range of causes in the differential diagnosis, including:
    - Urinary tract infection
    - PID
    - Pregnancy, especially ectopic
    - Ovarian cysts
    - Cancer
    - Vaginitis
    - Sexually transmitted infections
    - Gastrointestinal causes
    - Appendicitis
    - Muscle strain
    - Trauma

3. Percussion for abnormal air, masses, liver, spleen, costovertebral tenderness
4. Light palpation for tenderness, including rebound (pain after releasing pressure)
5. Deeper palpation for liver, masses, and unusual tenderness

ESSENTIAL FACTS

If you suspect severe pain or a mass, do not deeply palpate as this may cause rupture of an ovarian cyst, ectopic pregnancy, or appendix, if inflamed (appendicitis).

References

Carcio, H. A., & Secor, M. C. (2015). *Advanced health assessment of women: Clinical skills and procedures* (3rd ed., pp. 56–57). New York, NY: Springer Publishing.

Rhoads, J. (2006). *Advanced health assessment and diagnostic reasoning*. Philadelphia, PA: Lippincott Williams & Wilkins.

3

The Vulvar Exam

R. Mimi Secor

Performing a comprehensive assessment of the female external genitalia requires knowledge of the anatomy. A systemic approach is used to carefully observe and palpate the various tissues and anatomic features. Examining the vulvar region provides the opportunity to detect anatomic changes and other abnormal physical examination findings that may provide diagnostic clues about the possible diagnosis of any symptoms described during the interview.

In this chapter, you will learn how to:

- Describe the anatomy of the external genitalia, including key structures and landmarks
- Conduct a systematic assessment of the external genitalia
- Describe normal and abnormal external genitalia findings

THE APPROACH

After helping the woman assume the lithotomy position, offer her a self-examination mirror. Utilizing an adjustable telescoping mirror allows patient viewing without interference as the clinician conducts the examination. Some general strategies that help to reduce her anxiety include:

- Obtain the woman's permission before proceeding with the exam.
- Explain the steps involved in the exam and what the woman can expect to experience. This provides the woman with anticipatory guidance, education, and support.
- Answer questions as they arise; describing normal and abnormal findings to the woman is educational and often empowering.
- Wear gloves throughout the gynaecologic exam and when handling any equipment, supplies, or specimens.
- Use a cotton, Dacron, or new vaginal pH swab (VS-Sense) as a pointer to educate the woman about normal and abnormal anatomy and findings. This same swab may be used to separate skin folds and to assess for tenderness and allodynia (abnormal tenderness or pain to light touch).
- After the exam, don new gloves while handling lab specimens, including Papanicolaou (Pap) smears, sexually transmitted infection (STI; Table 3.1), and vaginal microscopy specimens.

ESSENTIAL FACTS

Some authorities recommend double gloving, then after performing the vulvar exam (Table 3.2), removing the outer glove in order to maintain an uncontaminated environment. When in doubt, it is better to change gloves than to risk contamination.

EXTERNAL EXAMINATION OF THE GENITALIA

The systematic approach to examining the external genitalia (Figure 3.1) includes an initial visual examination followed by palpation and separation of skin folds; assessment for tenderness, masses, muscle tension, or any other abnormal findings.

The systematic steps in the external examination are as follows:

- Visually inspect the suprapubic area, visualizing superiorly to inferiorly and then laterally

Table 3.1

Sexually Transmitted Infection Assessment of the Female

Infection + cause	Prevalence	Symptoms	Diagnosis
Chancroid *Haemophilus ducreyi*, Gram-negative bacillus	More common in sex trade	Women often asymptomatic	Culture positive for *H. ducreyi*, rule out more common HSV, also HIV, syphilis by RPR
Chlamydia Obligate intracellular parasite susceptible to antibiotics	Most common reported STI, 3 million new cases a year	Women often asymptomatic	Universal screening if <25 years old; urine polymerase chain reaction (PCR) or cervical testing; vaginal testing PCR or NAAT testing both approved
Genital herpes Type 1 or 2 herpes virus: both can infect genitals	Estimated 55 million Americans infected	Most asymptomatic; symptoms may include painful genital lesions, first infection most severe, recurrences most common with HSV 2, widely variable symptoms	If classic symptoms suspect HSV; culture if lesions, PCR culture more sensitive, expensive; type-specific serology IgG/HerpesSelect, 98% seroconversion 4 months post-HSV acquisition
Genital warts Noncogenic HPV 6, 11	1 million visits yearly, HPV affecting up to 80% of sexually active young women in the United States	Single or multiple, soft, fleshy, nontender, cauliflower-like lesions in genital area (vulvovaginal, anal, or cervix)	By exam, RPR to rule out condylomata lata of syphilis; colposcopy and/or biopsy of atypical lesions
Gonorrhea *Neisseria gonorrhoeae*, Gram-negative diplococcus bacteria	Second most common STI in the United States, especially among MSM	Women commonly asymptomatic, or abnormal vaginal discharge, dysuria, abnormal menses	Gram stain, culture, NAAT of cervical secretions; urine NAAT an option, too; vaginal NAAT for oropharyngeal testing

(continued)

Table 3.1

Sexually Transmitted Infection Assessment of the Female (continued)

Infection + cause	Prevalence	Symptoms	Diagnosis
Pelvic inflammatory disease Polymicrobial, various combinations, *N. gonorrhoeae*, *Chlamydia trachomatis*, anaerobes, and others	1 million new cases yearly, leading cause of female infertility	Many have no or atypical symptoms; symptoms include pain/tenderness in lower abdomen, uterus, ovaries, fever, chills, and elevated WBCs/erythrocyte sedimentation rate associated with menses	High index of suspicion, low threshold for diagnosis, positive cultures, Centers for Disease Control and Prevention criteria, pelvic exam tenderness, mucopus, WBCs on vaginal microscopy, gonorrhea, chlamydia or anaerobes/facultative bacteria
Syphilis *Treponema palladium* spirochete	Increasing among MSM, unusual in women, unless risk factors, higher rates in sex workers	Primary: classic chancre is painless, indurated ulcer in genital area, may evade diagnosis if vaginal Secondary: variable skin rash, may involve palmar hands, soles of feet Latent: few clinical symptoms, CNS changes	Primary: dark-field exam of chancre, with RPR serology Secondary/latent: RPR serology
Trichomoniasis Motile protozoan	Most common curable STI, 3 million U.S. women infected yearly; may be asymptomatic for years	Excessive, frothy, yellow-green vaginal discharge, exam findings variable, sometimes with genital erythema, swelling, and pruritus	Vaginal microscopy for typical motile trichomonads and WBCs; Pap should be verified with culture or microscopy Various vaginal cultures may also be used

CNS, central nervous system; HPV, human papillomavirus; HSV, herpes simplex virus; IgG, immunoglobulin G; MSM, men who have sex with men; NAAT, nucleic acid amplification testing; Pap, Papanicolaou; RPR, rapid plasma regain; STI, sexually transmitted infection, WBCs, white blood cells.

Source: Adapted with permission from Carcio and Secor (2010).

Table 3.2

Assessment of the Vulvar Region External Genitalia

Normal findings of area assessed	Abnormal: list findings, then conditions; need to be consistent
Vulva Labia majora—hair covered Labia minora—pink, moist, shiny Butterfly wing shape bilaterally	*Lesions*: biopsy if new, changing or suspicious, or persisting beyond 6 to 8 weeks (general guideline) Small nontender, nonpigmented nodules (Fordyce spots, normal variant, usually within Hart's line, inner labia) Nontender, firm, larger nodules (sebaceous cysts) Large, tender, swollen lump at 5 or 7 o'clock of introitus (Bartholin cyst) Single-stalk, finger-like tiny papules, inner labia (micropapillomatosis labialis, considered normal variant) Cauliflower-like growths, usually nontender (genital warts) Round, firm, umbilicated nontender papules (*Molluscum contagiosum*) Ulcer, nontender, fairly well-demarcated border (chancre of primary syphilis or chancroid) Single/clustered, tender vesicles or ulcerations (genital herpes, cellulitis, MRSA, hydradenitis suppurativa, trichomoniasis ulcers, HIV ulcers) Irregular, nontender, lesions; pigmented, red, or white (vulvar carcinoma/VIN, precancer) Scarring (genital mutilation/cutting, Crohn's disease, episiotomy, etc.) Distended blood vessels; tender, often in clusters (varicosities usually pregnancy related) Fissures: thin, tender, longitudinal (may be associated with infections [i.e., yeast or genital herpes], inflammation [i.e., allergic/contact reactions], skin conditions [i.e., LS, LSC) Fissures: large, tender, "knife-like lesions" (Crohn's disease)

(continued)

Table 3.2

Assessment of the Vulvar Region External Genitalia (continued)

Normal findings of area assessed	Abnormal: list findings, then conditions; need to be consistent
	Redness/erythema/tenderness Inflammation (seborrheic dermatitis, psoriasis, eczema, LP, allergens, irritants such as soaps, detergents, dryer sheets, chlorine) Infection (*Candida*, trichomoniasis, fungal, bacterial) Focal erythema may be associated with genital herpes, vestibulodynia if within the introital area/vestibule May be associated with acute, chronic vaginitis, or may be idiopathic *Discoloration or pigmentation* Dark or pigmented lesions (usually benign; but nevi can develop into melanoma); biopsy new, very dark, large, changing, or symptomatic lesions to rule out melanoma and other cancers/precancers White or hypopigmented areas (LS, squamous hyperplasia, also known as LSC, or possibly VIN) *Bruises* (consider possible sexual assault) *Anatomic changes associated with skin conditions* Flattening of the posterior labia minora (early LP) Loss of landmarks (LS, LP), agglutination (LS), flattening of labia (LS, LP), parchment-like changes (LS), tenderness, whitening (LS, LP, LSC biopsy is a must to clarify diagnosis and to rule out VIN, infection, irritant, contact, atrophy)

Clitoris
Round, pink, erectile tissue underneath the clitoral hood; size = approximately 2 cm (0.75 in.) × 0.5 cm (0.195 in.)

Enlargement
Masculinizing conditions (excess testosterone; use of testosterone-containing medications)
Atrophy
May virtually disappear (LS)

Urethral meatus
Pink tissue without discharge

Caruncle—small protrusion through the orifice that resembles a polyp (estrogen deprivation)
Prolapse of urethral mucosa—presents as a swollen red ring around the urinary meatus (menopause)
Leaking of urine—stress, urge, mixed incontinence

Vaginal introitus
Small amount of white to clear discharge
Intact hymen or hymenal tags/tissues
No bulging
No redness, lesions, tenderness, normal

Discharge (vaginitis; cervicitis)
Thick, pink membrane (imperforate hymen)
Anterior bulging (cystocele; may be aggravated by obesity)
Posterior bulging (rectocele, enterocele)
Focal erythema and tenderness at 5 and/or 7 o'clock (vestibulodynia)
Allodynia (suggests vestibulodynia)
Leaking of urine or feces (vaginal fistula)

Perineum and anus
Skin between vaginal introitus and anus should appear pink, smooth

Scar—episiotomy
Skin tags
Fissures
Erythema (vulvovaginitis)
Focal erythema in fourchette (vestibulodynia)
Hemorrhoids

LP, lichen planus; LS, lichen sclerosis; LSC, lichen simplex chronicus; MRSA, methicillin-resistant *Staphylococcus aureus*; VIN, vulvar intraepithelial neoplasia.
Source: Adapted with permission from Carcio and Secor (2015).

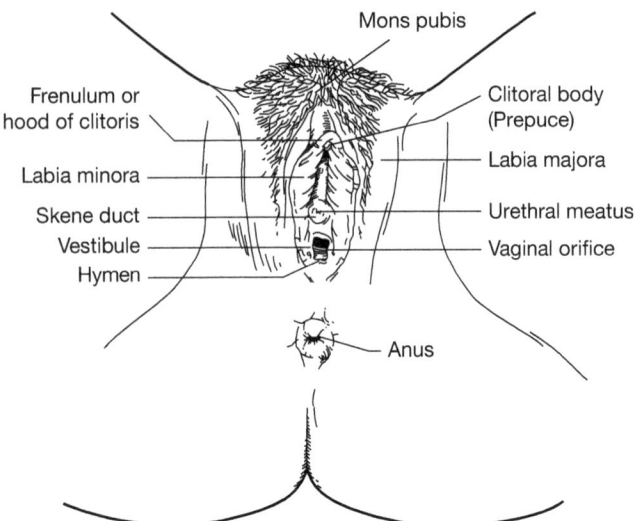

Figure 3.1 External genitalia (with revised labels). *Source: Carcio and Secor (2015).*

- Inspect the mons pubis for condition of skin and pubic hair or presence of lesions, masses, foreign bodies such as pubic lice, and/or tenderness
- Assess the clitoral hood, clitoris, urethral meatus, Skene's ducts adjacent to the urethral meatus, and the vaginal introitus
- Carefully examine the hymenal tissues, labia minora, labia majora, perineum, rectum, and sacrum areas
- Inspect and gently palpate the upper inner thighs, buttocks, and lower back depending on the woman's history and symptoms

FOCUS OF THE VISUAL EXAMINATION

Observe the vaginal introitus. The labia minora normally are shaped like butterfly wings. In early lichen planus (LP), there may be flattening or an absence of the lower posterior aspects of the labia minora. These findings may be symmetrical or asymmetrical. Observe for appearance of a cystocele (bulging or herniation of the bladder into the vagina and introitus) or rectocele (bulging of the rectum into the floor of the vagina).

Locate Hart's line, which is the mucocutaneous border separating the inner labia minora (pink, moist, thin, no hair) from the more keratinized skin lateral to the inner labia minora (normal skin color, thicker, hair covered). Hart's line extends superiorly to the clitoris and inferiorly to the perineum. Most women with vulvovaginitis are most symptomatic medial to Hart's line.

Identify the hymenal area. An imperforate hymen is a continuous membranous "fold" covering the vaginal introitus; a perforated hymen appears as multiple overlapping skin flaps along the margins of the introitus (more typically referred to as hymenal remnants). A hymen that appears imperforated (intact) is common in young girls and in virginal women.

Observe for abnormal findings in the genital area, which may include redness, swelling, tenderness, loss of landmarks, masses, foreign bodies such as pubic lice, lesions (such as vesicles, papules, or rashes), fissures, scarring, whitening, abnormal dark-pigmented lesions, agglutination of skin folds (the clinician should be able to separate skin folds), and absence of normal hair distribution.

Note any clinical signs indicating possible dermatologic conditions, including lesions, infections, or other abnormalities. Many clinicians and women assume most vulvovaginal complaints are related to "yeast," candida, or monilial infections. However, there are many nonyeast causes of vulvovaginal complaints, including vaginal causes (STIs, bacterial vaginosis [BV], atrophic changes), vulvar dermatologic conditions (lichen simplex chronicus, lichen sclerosis [LS], LP, sensitive skin, and conditions secondary to numerous possible external irritants), hygienic practices, and, less commonly, allergens.

Patient education tips: General vulvar self-care guidelines that the clinician can use to educate women are described in Appendix D.

Common STIs include the following:

- Chlamydia
- Herpes simplex (Figure 3.2a)
- Condylomata (genital warts; Figure 3.2b)
- Gonorrhea
- Pelvic inflammatory disease (PID)
- Syphilis
- Chancroid

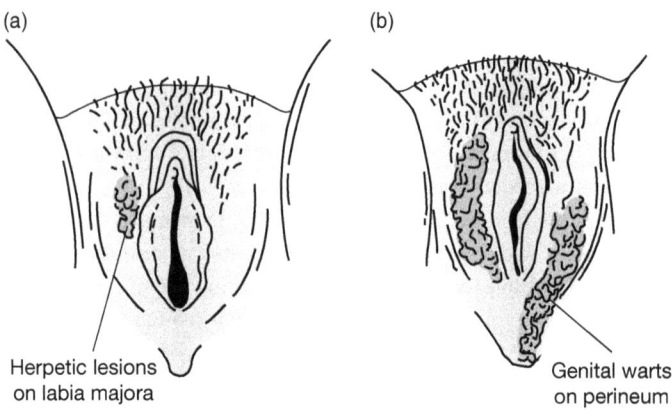

Figure 3.2 (a) Genital herpes. (b) Genital warts.

To complete the visual exam, palpation is required to separate skin folds; identify hidden clinical findings; and determine any areas of erythema, masses, or other abnormal skin findings. Palpation detects masses and tenderness not otherwise identified by inspection alone, such as Bartholin's gland cysts (Figure 3.3a, 3.3b). Use a cotton or Dacron swab to localize and grade tenderness and to assess for allodynia (abnormal sensation).

ESSENTIAL FACTS

Allodynia is the perception of tenderness or pain with light palpation in an area that is not normally painful when touched lightly with a gloved finger or a small swab. Allodynia may be associated with acute or chronic vulvar pain and/or vestibulodynia, vaginismus, and, less commonly, some dermatologic conditions such as LP or LS.

PALPATION

After completing the visual inspection of the vaginal introitus, separate the tissue fragments of the hymen (looking for focal erythema or lesions) and folds of the labia. Palpate the introitus for tenderness or masses, focusing on the Bartholin's gland duct areas, which are located

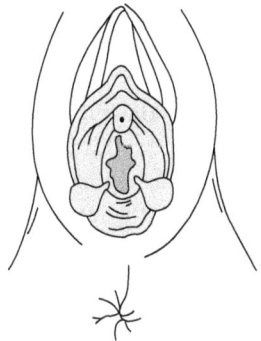

Figure 3.3(a) Bartholin's glands.

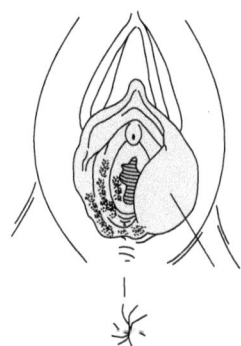

Figure 3.3(b) Bartholin cyst.

at 5 and 7 o'clock. Bartholin's glands should be smooth and nontender. Tenderness on palpation or presence of a mass requires follow-up. If tenderness is elicited, the location is recorded as if the introitus is a face of a clock (e.g., erythema at 3 o'clock) and the severity of tenderness rated on a scale of 1 to 10 (with 10 representing the most severe pain).

Next, assess for vaginal introital tone and laxity.

- Abnormal tone may be referred to as *hytone dysfunction* and may be more marked on one side than the other.
- Vaginismus, the involuntary spasm of the pelvic floor muscles, is usually associated with anxiety and possibly a past history of sexual trauma. Examining a woman with vaginismus can be very challenging and is discussed in Part II.

When evaluating vaginal introital tone, perform the following maneuvers to test for laxity and tone:

- The test for laxity involves asking the women to bear down, or perform the Valsalva maneuver; this may expose a cystocele, bulging of the bladder into the vagina (Figure 3.4), or a rectocele, bulging of the rectum up into the vaginal floor (Figure 3.5).
- Before and during the Valsalva maneuver, observe for prolapse of the uterus (a descent of the uterus from its normal position into the vagina, and sometimes out of the body). Uterine prolapse (Figure 3.6) may also be apparent without the pressure placed upon it during the Valsalva maneuver. If present, note the degree of prolapse from first degree (minimal lowering of cervix into vagina cavity), second degree (where the cervix is visible at the vaginal introitus), third degree (where the cervix is visible outside

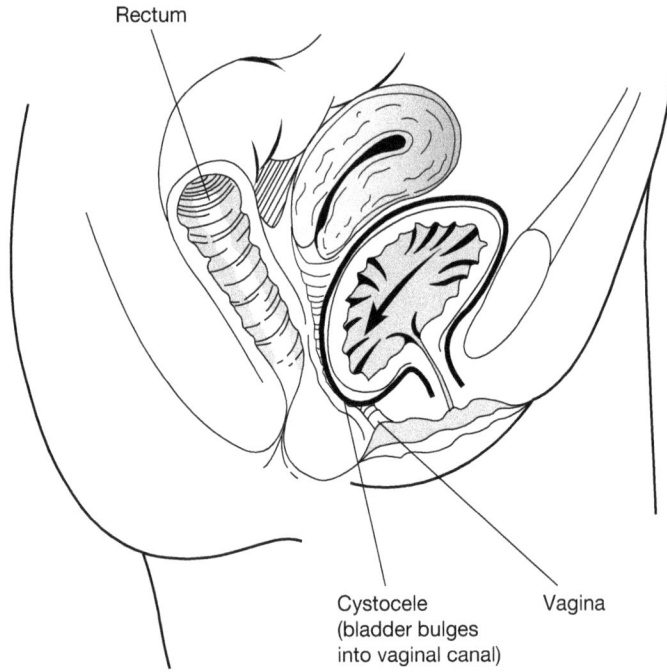

Figure 3.4 Cystocele.

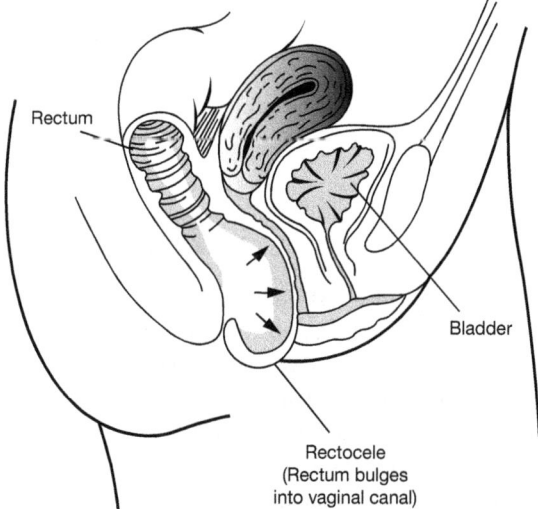

Figure 3.5 Rectocele.

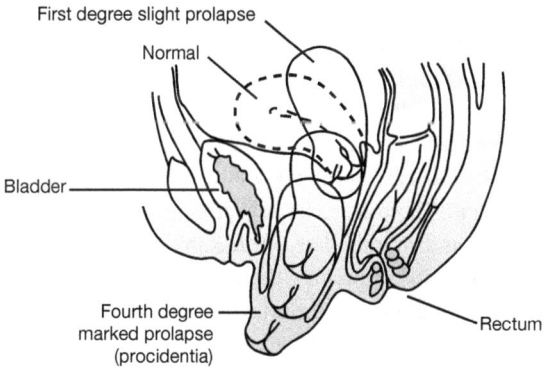

Figure 3.6 Degrees of uterine prolapse.

the vagina), and fourth degree (where the cervix and the uterus are entirely externally prolapsed). This most extreme case is called *procidentia*.

- The test for introital tone, or hytone dysfunction, involves palpating the introital tissues for abnormal muscle tension/spasm and associated tenderness. Introital tone is also assessed by inserting one finger into the vagina and asking the women to "tighten" around the clinician's finger. This requires contracting the pubococcygeal (PC) muscle as though she is holding her urine and/or bowels.

ESSENTIAL FACTS

A positive "sticky glove test" indicates possible atrophic vaginitis. This test is conducted by lightly palpating the inner labia minora and noting whether your gloved fingers adhere to the tissue. This finding is common in postmenopausal women, due to diminished estrogen production. The finding is subtle and the inexperienced clinician must be attentive to appreciate it. (See Chapter 11 for more information on atrophic vaginitis.)

PELVIC FLOOR REHABILITATION

- Some women may not be able to isolate the PC muscle. Women who are experiencing symptoms of overactive bladder (OAB), including urgency, frequency, or leakage; dyspareunia; or chronic vulvar pain may benefit from pelvic floor rehabilitation combined with biofeedback and possibly electrical stimulation (also called *E-stim*). These exercises help strengthen the pelvic floor (Figure 3.7) and counter detrusor instability associated with OAB, often greatly improving the symptoms of OAB.
- Pelvic floor rehabilitation includes exercises to strengthen the pelvic floor muscles (levator ani and PC muscles). These exercises include Kegels (5–10 seconds) and "quick flick" (5 seconds) exercises.
- E-stim helps women isolate and learn how to contract their PC muscle, which is required to perform both Kegel's and quick-flick exercises.

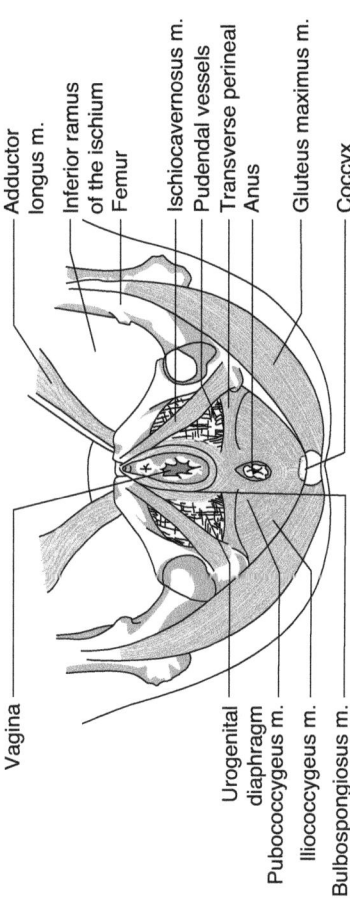

Figure 3.7 Anatomy and musculature of pelvic floor. m, muscle.

References

Carcio, H. A., & Secor, M. C. (2010). *Advanced health assessment of women: Clinical skills and procedures* (2nd ed., pp. 340–342). New York, NY: Springer Publishing.

Carcio, H. A., & Secor, M. C. (2015). *Advanced health assessment of women: Clinical skills and procedures* (3rd ed., pp. 67–69). New York, NY: Springer Publishing.

4

The Speculum Exam

R. Mimi Secor

The purpose of the speculum exam is to visualize the vagina and the cervix. Note both normal findings and abnormalities. The speculum exam also allows the examiner to collect a cervical sample for a Papanicolaou (Pap) smear and to screen for sexually transmitted infections (STIs), as well as vaginitis as indicated. To optimize the results of the testing, the sample must be collected properly. (Cervical cancer screening guidelines appear in Table 4.1.)

In this chapter, you will learn how to:

- Prepare for the speculum exam
- Select the appropriate speculum for an individual woman
- Insert, secure, and remove the speculum
- Locate and visualize the cervix and properly obtain a Pap smear

PREPARING TO PERFORM THE SPECULUM EXAM

Gather the equipment needed to perform the exam:

- A light suitable for illuminating the pelvic area during the exam; consider using a gooseneck light or a light attached to a plastic speculum

Table 4.1

The 2012 Cervical Cancer Screening Guidelines	
Age 21	Screening should begin
Ages 21–29	Cytology alone is recommended every 3 years
Age 25–65	hr-HPV every 3 years with reflex cytology (Huh et al., 2015)
Ages 30–65	Cotesting (Pap and HPV) every 5 years is recommended
	If HPV testing is not available, cytology alone should be continued every 3 years
Age 65	Screening may stop

HPV, human papillomavirus; hr-HPV, high-risk human papillomavirus.
Source: Saslow et al. (2012).

- Vaginal speculum: both plastic and metal are suitable options
- Water-soluble lubricant
- Supplies for obtaining the Pap smear and any cultures that may be necessary
- Nonlatex gloves

PREPARE THE WOMAN FOR WHAT TO EXPECT DURING THE SPECULUM EXAM

The following hints are useful in promoting comfort and reducing anxiety (reprinted with permission from Carcio & Secor, 2010, p. 62):

- Offer an educational pelvic examination by explaining the techniques used, the sensations that the woman may feel, and the function of the body parts examined.
- Explain each aspect of the examination as it is performed, to reduce the woman's level of anxiety. Always be as gentle as possible.
- Explain the rationale for each aspect of the exam and provide clues about what she might "feel"; for example, "You might feel some pressure when I insert my fingers into your vagina."
- Suggest coping strategies to minimize stress she might be experiencing:

- Encourage her to progressively relax different body parts or to take deep breaths and exhale slowly at any point during the exam when she feels especially tense.
- Teach use of "self-talk" statements, such as "I know this may be slightly uncomfortable but I will be fine."
- Reassure her that you (the examiner) will stop the exam at any time that she becomes uncomfortable or asks you to stop the exam.

POSITIONING THE WOMAN

The lithotomy position is the traditional position for the vaginal or speculum exam. Assist the woman to slide down to the end of the examination table while providing support. This can be done by placing your hands at the end of the table while asking the patient to slide down until they bump into your hands. This ensures the woman knows when she has reached the end of the table/has slid down far enough, and also helps her feel more comfortable and secure. When she is in the correct position, her buttocks should be at the end of the examination table (slightly overhanging), with her heels placed in the stirrups, knees bent, and hips externally rotated and abducted.

Inform the woman prior to inserting the speculum, explain the procedure, and remind her of the sensations she may experience during each part of the procedure. Ask the woman to inform you at any time of pain or other unpleasant symptoms experienced during the exam, and assure her that the examination will stop at any time if she so requests.

SELECTING THE SPECULUM

Vaginal specula are available in both metal and plastic of varying styles, sizes, and quality. Plastic specula come in fewer sizes, styles, and, most important, they range in quality. The less expensive plastic specula may not reliably unlock prior to removal. This inability to release the speculum can cause the clinician anxiety and the woman additional anxiety, pain, and possibly injury when the clinician removes the speculum with the blades in an open position. To lessen this risk, the clinician should be familiar with the speculum prior to the examination; the examiner might consider holding the blades open and not locking it in place.

The major advantages of metal specula include the following:

- Available in many styles (Pederson, Graves, bariatric, and many others)
- Available in many sizes (small, medium, large, etc.) to accommodate different types of women and their unique needs, including pediatric, multiparous, obese, and those with physical disabilities
- Can be prewarmed with tap water, by holding the speculum briefly in gloved hands, by placing it on a heating pad (on low setting in the exam table storage drawer), or by running the speculum under warm water
- Can be sterilized for reuse, offering an economical and "green" option

The major advantages of plastic specula include the following:

- Plastic specula provide an unobstructed view of the vaginal walls through the clear blades.
- No prewarming of the speculum before insertion is required.
- Use may reduce her anxiety because the clear plastic appearance is less "scary" than metal.
- Some models are designed with plug-in lighting systems (such as Welch Allyn corded or cordless) and offer enhanced illumination and examination of the vagina and cervix.
- Conveniently, this external light source may also be used to examine the vulva prior to speculum insertion.

On occasion, plastic specula can break in situ or be difficult to "unlock" upon removal. This is potentially traumatic for both the woman and the clinician. If the speculum cannot be unlocked, then it must be removed with the blades open, possibly causing pain and injuring the woman's external genitalia. Another disadvantage of plastic specula is their contribution to medical waste because they are not reusable.

Appropriate Speculum Size

To determine the size and type of the speculum most appropriate for examining a woman, the clinician should evaluate the diameter and tone of the vaginal introitus. For symptomatic or anxious women, the clinician should consider using a smaller speculum.

Helpful tips to reduce discomfort during the exam include the following:

- Palpate the cervix before inserting the speculum, especially if this is her first exam, if the woman is symptomatic, if she has a history of abuse or trauma, or if she has experienced "difficult or challenging" exams in the past.
- Use a small amount of lubricant if needed.
- Palpating the cervix in advance of the speculum exam may help in selecting the more appropriate speculum style and/or size.

INSERTING THE SPECULUM

- Separate the labia minora with your nondominant hand to expose the vaginal opening.
- Hold the speculum with your dominant hand, grasping it in a manner that keeps the blades securely closed. To do this, place your index finger on top of the upper blade near the handle, and your middle finger under the base of the lower blade (where the handle meets the blades). This is the recommended hand position for insertion and removal of the speculum.
- Holding the speculum at a slight sideways angle, insert the speculum in a downward direction, approximately 2 inches into the vagina (see Figure 4.1a).
- Use a gentle side-to-side "shimmy" to advance the speculum.
- When the speculum is in place, open the speculum by repositioning both hands: one hand controls opening the speculum blades and the other hand holds the lower handle of the speculum (see Figure 4.1b).
- Once partially visualized, open the speculum more until the cervix pops fully into view (Figure 4.1c). You may have to lift the lower "chin" of the cervix with a further gentle side-to-side "shimmy" of the speculum blades to "coax" the cervix into full view.
- Secure the speculum by either rotating the metal wheel/knob on the side of the speculum handle or locking the plastic blades together in an open position, just enough to view and sample the cervix.

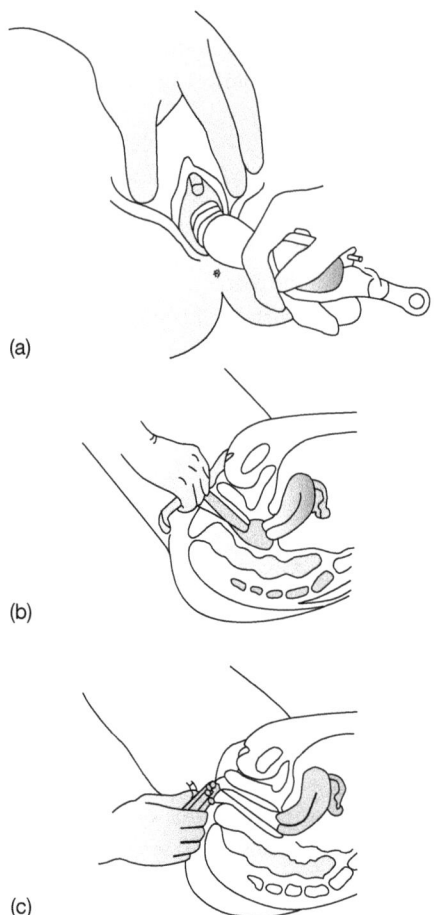

Figure 4.1 Speculum insertion. (a) Position index finger and thumb on the top, place the middle and ring finger under the lower speculum blade (see the description in the text). (b) Turn the speculum so that the blades are horizontal to the examining table while advancing the speculum into the vagina, pressing downward with the lower blade on the posterior vaginal wall at a 45-degree angle. (c) Once in place, open the speculum and maneuver the blades until the cervix is visible.

Potential discomfort occurs from tension at the vaginal opening caused by opening the speculum blades. Larger specula create more tension or stretching of the vaginal opening and potentially cause more discomfort. This is especially important to remember when examining symptomatic women; those undergoing their first examination; pediatric patients; and any women with a history of anxiety, vaginismus, dyspareunia, or emotional or physical sexual abuse or pain.

ESSENTIAL FACTS

- To examine certain women who are symptomatic, anxious, or have a history of sexual abuse, it may be necessary to open the speculum blades only partially, while viewing and sampling the cervix as quickly as possible.
- When using a plastic Welch Allyn speculum, take care to lift the adjustment tab (white ratchet) when opening the speculum blades to avoid causing a loud repetitive clicking sound as the blades are opened. If you do not lift the tab, you should warn the woman to expect this "clicking" sound.

INSPECTING THE VAGINA AND CERVIX

Visualize the vagina for color (normally pink) and rugations, which are vaginal folds normally present in women of reproductive age. The clinician may note a small amount of opaque, white, nonmalodorous discharge. During the visual inspection, the clinician should also note any redness, pallor, lack of rugation, abnormal bulging of the vaginal walls (a cystocele is a bulging of the upper front wall of the vagina, a rectocele is a bulging of the lower rear wall of the vagina, and an enterocele is a bulging of the upper rear wall of the vagina), lesions, abnormal discharge (such as frothy, yellow, or malodorous discharge), lesions, foreign bodies, or other unusual findings (Table 4.2 and Figure 4.2).

The cervix is normally pink, smooth, and nontender, with clear mucus noted at the os. A cervix that is blue-tinged (cyanotic in appearance) indicates possible pregnancy. A nulliparous os is oval or round; a parous os is slit-like (Figure 4.3). Abnormalities may include the presence of redness, friability, tenderness, lesions, and abnormal cervical mucus.

Table 4.2

Normal and Abnormal Assessment Findings of the Vagina and Cervix

Findings of area assessed

Normal	Abnormal
Vagina	
Normally pink	Gonorrhea or chlamydia: abundance of polymorphonuclear WBCs
Discharge: opaque, white, nonmalodorous mucus emitted from Skene's glands	Vaginal discharge: ■ Candida vulvovaginitis: thick, white, clumpy discharge ■ Bacterial vaginosis: thin, fishy odor, adherent, homogeneous white or gray ■ Trichomoniasis: yellow, grayish-green, frothy, malodorous
Normal pH: acidic	
Vagina: mucosa Normal: rugae (mucosal folds) negative	Atrophic vaginitis; thin, pale, atrophic-appearing mucosa, variable discharge, scant, copious, watery, yellow; lack of rugae is evidence of low estrogen level ■ Cystocele: bulging (herniation) of the bladder into the upper front vaginal wall ■ Rectocele: bulging (herniation) of the rectum into the rear vaginal wall ■ Enterocele: bulging (herniation) of the small intestine into the upper rear vaginal wall
Cervix	
Size and shape Nulliparous (small and oval or round) Parous (slit-like)	Laceration or tears: may result from a precipitous delivery; tiny os (may also be noted in nulliparous women who are not taking estrogen)
Surface: color is pink, smooth, soft, mobile, and nontender on movement	Bluish (cyanotic): associated with pregnancy Tender on movement: may indicate pelvic inflammatory disease Fixed or immobile: may indicate endometriosis or a tumor Polyps: small, red-purple, pedunculated protrusions; typically arising from endocervical canal; more common during menstruating years and in parous women in fifth decade Nabothian cysts: can be single or multiple; small, translucent or yellow nodules on the cervical surface

(continued)

Table 4.2

Normal and Abnormal Assessment Findings of the Vagina and Cervix (*continued*)

Findings of area assessed

Normal	Abnormal
Mucosa characteristics: intact, no lesions	Friability: may be related to infection such as chlamydia or vaginitis
	Wart-like excoriation: may be associated with cervical cancer
	Extension of endocervical columnar epithelium on the ectocervix (ectropion): evidence of increased estrogen production in pregnancy or effect of birth control pills
	Erosion: friable tissues surrounding os-associated cervicitis
Location	Lower in the vagina: possible uterine prolapse
	Lowering of more than 3 cm may suggest an ovarian mass

WBC, white blood cell.

Sources: Carcio and Secor (2010), Rhoads (2006).

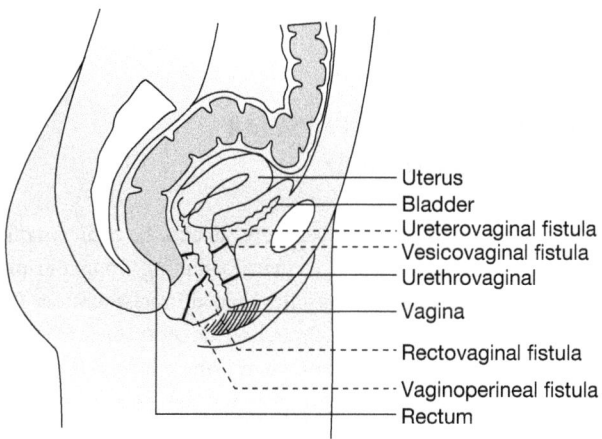

Figure 4.2 Locations of various fistulas.

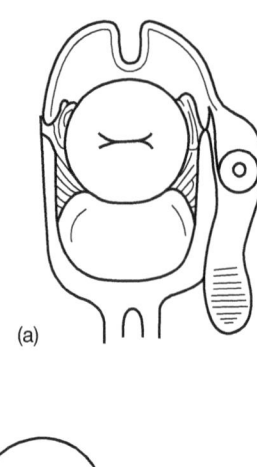

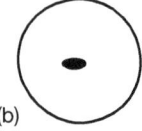

Figure 4.3 Inspecting the cervix. (a) Multiparous cervix. (b) Nulliparous cervix.

ESSENTIAL FACTS

If a visible lesion is noted on the cervix, a colposcopy is recommended regardless of the Pap smear result. This is important even and especially if the Pap smear report is negative.

COLLECTING THE CERVICAL PAP SMEAR (AND OPTIONAL STI TESTING)

Sample the ectocervix, or outer cervix (visible to the clinician during the speculum exam), with either a cervical sampling broom or a plastic spatula. Carry out sampling in a smooth, continuous manner (without disconnecting from the cervix), circling the cervix once when using the spatula and three to five times when using a broom (Figure 4.4). The broom samples both the ectocervix and the endocervix simultaneously, so only one collection tool is needed when this device is used.

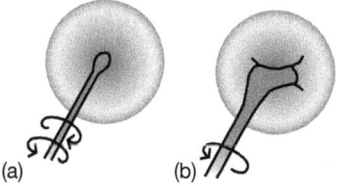

Figure 4.4 Pap smear collection technique. (a) Procedure for collecting endocervical sample for Pap smear and culture for gonorrhea and chlamydia testing using a Dacron swab or cytobrush: Insert the Dacron swab or cytobrush into the os and rotate a quarter to a half turn. Vigorously mix sample in vial of liquid. (b) Procedure for collecting ectocervical sample for Pap smear: Firmly place the longer projection of the notched end of the Ayre spatula into the os and rotate 360 degrees; hold the horizontal surface containing the sample in the upright position as you withdraw the spatula. Place the flat side of the spatula against the labeled glass slide and smear uniformly across the slide, using one firm motion.

ESSENTIAL FACTS

"Do it yourself Pap." With the cytobrush in position at the cervical os, ask the woman to cough. This causes the cervix to descend, resulting in the cervix "taking its own Pap smear" while simply rotating the cytobrush.

Place the sampling tools in the liquid-filled vial, rub the collection tools together, and mix vigorously. Next, remove the spatula and cytobrush collection tools from the vial and discard. When using the broom, swirl it vigorously in the vial, and then snap the broom tip off into the collection vial.

With the availability of various new commercial polymerase chain reaction (PCR), Pap/HPV (human papillomavirus)/STI/vaginitis testing systems (GenPath, Medical Diagnostic Laboratories [MDL], Quest, and others), it is now possible to collect one cervical or one cervicovaginal or lesion sample and obtain samples for multiple screening tests from this one collection. These new testing systems are quick, easy, accurate, and affordable and provide a convenient approach to testing in the context of the gynaecologic exam.

OTHER DIAGNOSTIC TESTS TO CONSIDER PERFORMING DURING THE SPECULUM EXAM

Conducting vaginal pH and amine/KOH (potassium hydroxide)/whiff testing and vaginal microscopy/wet mount/hanging drop should be considered if indicated based on history, risk factors, and exam findings. Exam findings that suggest further testing include abnormal vaginal discharge and/or the presence of lesions, rashes, or tenderness. The process of performing and documenting these tests is summarized in Appendices B and C.

The vaginal sample should carefully be obtained from the **lateral** vaginal wall using a plastic spatula (preferred) or a Dacron swab. Use care to avoid introducing cervical samples, as this mucus is more alkaline and can interfere with accurate vaginal pH testing. If vaginal pH or amine/KOH test results are abnormal, vaginal microscopy and/or STI vaginitis lab testing (PCR or non-PCR) should be considered. The differential diagnosis of vaginal infections is summarized in Table 4.3.

REMOVING THE SPECULUM

To loosen the speculum's "grip" on the cervix, open the speculum blades slightly while backing the speculum away from the cervix. This is especially important when removing a Welch Allyn speculum, which can be challenging to release from the cervix.

Once the speculum is free of the cervix, close the speculum blades and remove the speculum. Apply slight downward pressure to avoid traumatizing the clitoral area. On occasion, a non-Welch Allyn plastic speculum can be difficult to unlock. Unlocking the blades is required to close the speculum, allowing easy and painless removal.

ESSENTIAL FACTS

If you are unable to unlock and release the plastic speculum blades, try not to panic! Take a deep breath, ask the woman to cough forcefully, and quickly remove the open speculum. Try to avoid traumatizing the clitoral area while removing the speculum.

Table 4.3

Differential Diagnosis of Vaginal Infections

Condition	Vulvovaginal symptoms	Vaginal discharge	Lactobacilli	pH	Microscopy
Candida sp., yeast	Mild to severe itching and vulvovaginal erythema	Variable quality/quantity Classic: white, clumpy, "curd-like"	Variable	<4.7	KOH or saline Hyphae, pseudohyphae, and/or spores "spaghetti and meatballs"
Bacterial vaginosis	Variable; itching absent to mild Mild irritation Possible mild vulvovaginal erythema	Opaque, white, malodorous discharge, fishy odor, particularly after intercourse and with menses	Few	>4.6	Saline Clue cells Few WBCs, KOH/amine test positive
Trichomonas	Variable; mild to severe vulvar itching Petechiae of cervix "strawberry cervix"; vulvar erythema, ulceration	Variable quality/quantity Yellow-green May be frothy, malodorous	Variable	>4.6	Saline trichomonads Many WBCs KOH/amine test +/−
Atrophic vaginitis	Pruritus, irritation Vulvovaginal dryness and dyspareunia Smooth vaginal walls Few lactobacilli	Red, tender vulva and vagina Variable discharge, lack of rugae Few lactobacilli	Few	>4.6	Saline Parabasal cells WBCs variable, KOH/amine test negative
Desquamative inflammatory vaginitis	Erythema; diffuse or focal of vulva and vagina Pruritus, irritation, dyspareunia	Variable; yellow-green, may be copious No odor	Few	>4.6	Saline Many parabasal, basal cells Many WBCs, KOH/amine test negative Few lactobacilli

KOH, potassium hydroxide; WBCs, white blood cells.

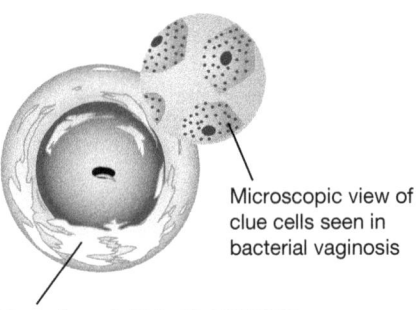

Microscopic view of clue cells seen in bacterial vaginosis

(a) View of cervix through speculum

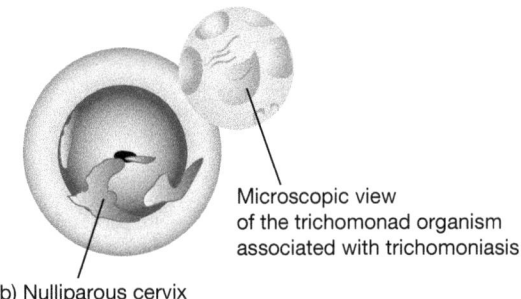

Microscopic view of the trichomonad organism associated with trichomoniasis

(b) Nulliparous cervix

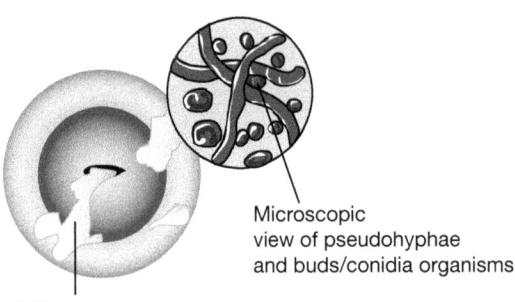

Microscopic view of pseudohyphae and buds/conidia organisms

(c) Multiparous cervix

Figure 4.5 (a) View of cervix through speculum. (b) Nulliparous cervix. (c) Multiparous cervix.

Exhibit 4.1

Sample Documentation of the Vulvar, Speculum, and Bimanual Portions of the Gynaecologic Exam

External genitalia: Normal distribution of pubic hair and normal anatomy; no masses, lesions, abnormal discharge, or tenderness; good muscle tone

Vagina: Pink; rugated without bulging or lesions; scant, opaque white discharge without odor; vaginal pH 4.0 (normal), amine/KOH test negative, vaginal microscopy negative for clue cells, trichomonads, yeast forms, or white blood cells (WBCs)

Cervix: Pink, smooth, no lesions or mucopus; nontender, no cervical motion tenderness (CMT)

DISCARDING THE SPECULUM

Plastic specula are for single use and should be properly discarded, and metal specula are sterilized/autoclaved and reused. Do not discard the speculum immediately as it may be needed to obtain additional vaginal samples for vaginal pH, amine/KOH testing, vaginal microscopy, or STI vaginitis testing (Figure 4.5).

References

Carcio, H. A., & Secor, M. C. (2010). *Advanced health assessment of women: Clinical skills and procedures* (2nd ed.). New York, NY: Springer Publishing.

Huh, W. K., Ault, K. A., Chelmow, D., Davey, D. D., Goulart, R. A., Garcia, F. A. R., . . . & Einstein, M. H. (2015). Use of primary high-risk human papillomavirus testing for cervical cancer screening: Interim clinical guidance. *Obstetrics & Gynecology, 125*(2), 330–337.

Rhoads, J. (2006). *Advanced health assessment and diagnostic reasoning.* Philadelphia, PA: Lippincott Williams & Wilkins.

Saslow, D., Solomon, D., Lawson, H. W., Killackey, M., Kulasingam, S. L., Cain, P., . . . ACS-ASCCP-ASCP Cervical Cancer Guideline Committee (2012). American Cancer Society, American Society for Colposcopy and Cervical Pathology, and American Society for Clinical Pathology screening guidelines for the prevention and early detection of cervical cancer. *CA: A Cancer Journal for Clinicians, 62*, 147–172. doi:10.3322 /caac.21139.

5

The Bimanual Exam

R. Mimi Secor

The bimanual exam allows the clinician to assess the vagina, cervix, uterus, and ovaries. It should be performed in a gentle but thorough manner, first palpating the vagina, then the uterus, ovaries, and, if indicated, the rectovaginal structures, and rectum last.

In this chapter, you will learn how to:

- Perform the bimanual examination for palpating the uterus and ovaries
- Perform a rectovaginal exam

The traditional approach is to perform the speculum exam prior to conducting the bimanual exam. However, some clinicians recommend conducting the bimanual exam prior to the speculum exam. Advantages to this sequence include less discomfort with the speculum exam, an opportunity to locate the cervix prior to speculum insertion, and less need for lubrication with the speculum exam.

> **ESSENTIAL FACTS**
>
> In women of reproductive age, you may not be able to palpate the ovaries during the bimanual examination. This is not cause for alarm, nor does it require additional testing unless the woman is symptomatic or high risk for ovarian cancer, or unless you suspect other conditions such as endometriosis. In contrast, if you palpate ovaries in a postmenopausal woman, consider this abnormal, and conduct a thorough workup to rule out pathology. Tests to consider include a transvaginal ultrasound, cancer antigen 125 (CA125) test, other tests as indicated, and referral to a gynaecologist.

THE BIMANUAL EXAM

The bimanual exam is conducted while standing at the foot of the examination table with the woman's buttocks at the end of the table. Place one gloved hand on the lower abdomen just above the mid-suprapubic area and, using a small amount of lubricant, insert one, or preferably two, gloved finger(s) into the vagina. Using lubricant reduces discomfort and facilitates the exam. Begin the bimanual exam by thoroughly palpating the vagina and cervix, noting areas of tenderness or masses.

To palpate the uterus, gently apply suprapubic pressure while positioning fingertips under the cervix and gently lifting up. Assess the uterus for position (angle), size, shape, contour, mobility, and tenderness. Note any abnormal findings such as tenderness (suggesting pelvic inflammatory disease [PID]), masses (suggesting fibroids), and lack of mobility (possible endometriosis).

The position of the uterus within the pelvis varies (see Figure 5.1). An anteverted uterus is angled toward the abdomen, whereas a retroverted uterus is angled toward the tailbone and rectum. Bimanual palpation of the anteverted uterus is shown in Figure 5.2.

A normal uterus is approximately the size of a lemon or small pear, but can range somewhat in size. The uterus is normally smooth, semi-firm, nontender, and mobile. If the uterus is tender, rule out PID. If the uterus is diffusely enlarged, rule out pregnancy and consider additional diagnostic testing based on the history, exam, and differential

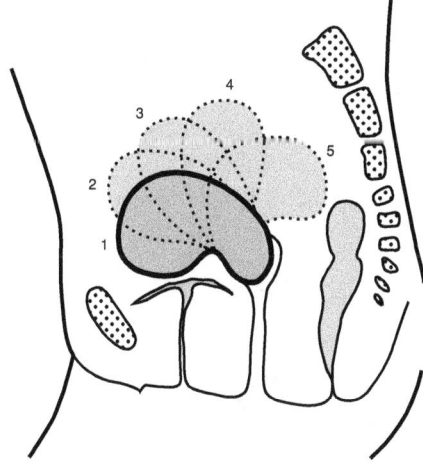

Figure 5.1 Positions of the uterus. (1) Anteflexed, (2) anteverted, (3) midposition, (4) retroverted, and (5) retroflexed. *Source: Carcio and Secor (2010).*

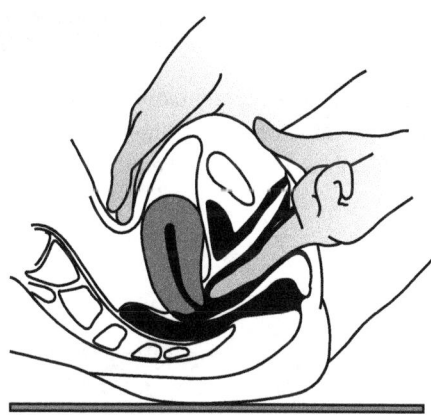

Figure 5.2 Bimanual palpation of the anteverted uterus. *Source: Carcio and Secor (2010).*

diagnosis. If the uterus is irregular and unusually firm, suspect fibroids and confirm with transvaginal ultrasound and/or hysteroscopy (Figure 5.3).

The uterus is not always easy to palpate, especially if the woman is obese, anxious, physically disabled, or elderly. Examining these special populations is discussed in Chapter 10.

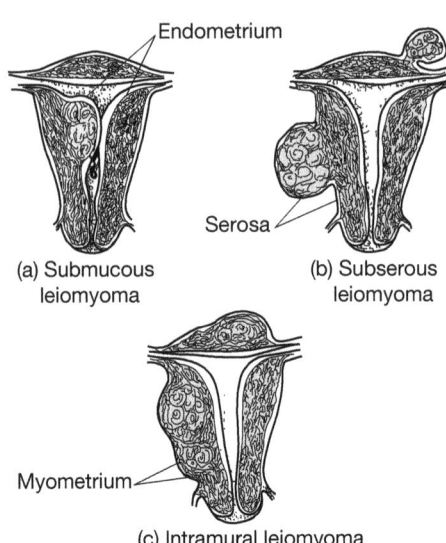

Figure 5.3 Appearance of uterine fibroids. *Source: Carcio and Secor (2010).*

ESSENTIAL FACTS

If the uterus is not palpable suprapubically, it may be retroverted, or "tipped" back toward the woman's tailbone. In this case, the uterus may be palpable only by rectovaginal exam (Figure 5.4).

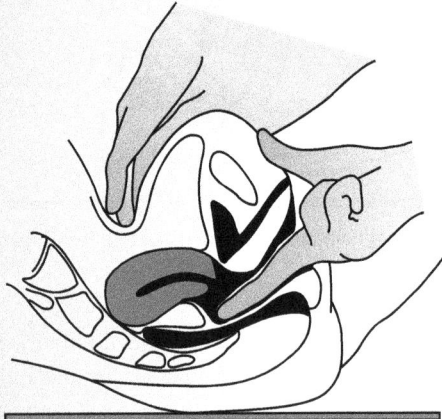

Figure 5.4 Bimanual palpation of the retroverted uterus. *Source: Carcio and Secor (2010).*

THE ADNEXAL EXAM

Perform the adnexal exam next. During this part of the exam, the clinician will examine the ovaries, which are located lateral to the fundus of the uterus and are about the size of almonds. Assess the ovaries for size (enlarged), shape (masses), and tenderness.

To examine the ovaries (Figure 5.5):

- Move abdominal hand to either the right or left lateral lower abdomen area, just lateral to the fundus of the uterus
- Position the fingers of the vaginal hand in the vaginal fornix of the adnexal side being examined
- Apply pressure similar to that used to palpate the uterus
- Repeat this same technique on the opposite side to examine the second ovary

Ovaries normally are almond sized, nontender, and semifirm (Table 5.1); however, it is not uncommon for them not to be palpable. Endometriosis may cause the ovaries to be located behind the uterus

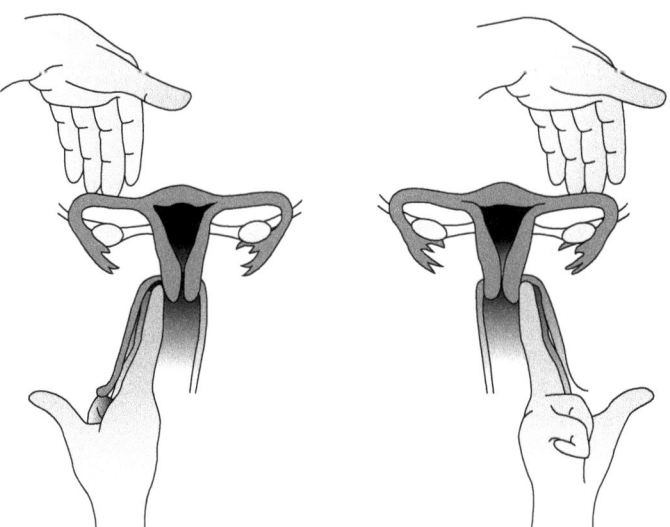

Figure 5.5 Bimanual examination of the ovaries and adnexae. *Sources: Carcio (1998); Gray (1980).*

Table 5.1

Assessment Findings of the Uterus and Adnexae: Normal and Abnormal

Findings of area assessed

Normal	Abnormal
Uterus	
Size: approximate size of a lemon	Enlargement: may indicate pregnancy or other mass
Normally smooth, semifirm, nontender, and mobile	Tender: possible pelvic inflammatory disease (PID) or endometriosis
	Irregular: may suggest fibroids
Position Most often anteverted, anteflexed (angled toward the abdomen) Freely movable	Retroverted, retroflexed (angled toward the tailbone) uterus may be difficult to palpate bimanually; a rectovaginal exam may be required; may be the result of endometriosis
Adnexae	
Ovaries Size: almond size Nontender, semifirm, and mobile	Enlargement: may be due to cystic enlargement, polycystic ovarian syndrome (PCOS), or tubal pregnancy; palpation will convey sense of "fullness"; may be tender; further testing is required to distinguish
	Endometriosis: may push ovaries to relocate behind the uterus, this position is called *holding hands*
Postmenopausal—usually not palpable	If palpable, consider abnormal and investigate
Fallopian tubes Normal: about 5 inches in length, rubbery, half the diameter of a pencil, not palpable, and nontender	If palpable, consider salpingitis or an ectopic pregnancy; in rare cases, may be associated with fallopian tube cancer
	If palpable and feel like fibrous bands, consider previous salpingitis or endometriosis

Source: Adapted from Carcio and Secor (2010); Rhoads (2006).

(referred to as *holding hands*), so they will not be palpable. Cystic enlargement of the ovaries will feel like fullness in the affected adnexal area and may be tender or nontender. A tubal pregnancy is indistinguishable clinically from an ovarian cyst, so additional testing is

Exhibit 5.1

Sample Documentation of the Vulvar, Speculum, and Bimanual Portions of the Gynaecologic Exam

External genitalia: Normal distribution of pubic hair and normal anatomy; no masses, lesions, abnormal discharge, or tenderness

Vagina: Pink; rugated without bulging or lesions; scant opaque white discharge without odor; good muscle tone; vaginal pH 4.0 (normal), amine/KOH (potassium hydroxide) test negative, vaginal microscopy negative for clue cells, trichomonads, yeast forms, or white blood cells (WBCs)

Cervix: Pink, smooth, no lesions, or mucopus; nontender, no cervical motion tenderness (CMT)

Uterus: Anteverted, normal size, shape, contour (NSSC), mobile, nontender, without palpable masses

Adnexae: Ovaries palpated, normal size, nontender, and no masses palpated

Rectovaginal: No lesions, masses, or fissures; nontender, small amount of brown soft stool present, guaiac test negative

---

urgently needed to determine the underlying etiology. This may include pelvic ultrasound, pregnancy testing, complete blood count (CBC) with differential, CA125, and a sedimentation rate. A history of unprotected intercourse and late menses increases the risk of pregnancy and the clinician's index of suspicion.

The ovaries may be palpable without conducting a rectovaginal exam, but when they are not palpable on the vaginal bimanual exam, the rectovaginal bimanual exam may be particularly helpful (see Chapter 6).

The fallopian tubes, considered part of the adnexae (Exhibit 5.1), are not typically palpable because of their small size. They are approximately 5 inches in length, about half the diameter of a pencil, and rubbery. If palpable, consider the possibility of salpingitis or endometriosis.

References

Carcio, H. A. (1998). *Management of the infertile woman* (p. 100). Philadelphia, PA: Lippincott-Raven.

Carcio, H. A., & Secor, M. C. (2010). *Advanced health assessment of women: Clinical skills and procedures* (2nd ed., p. 9). New York, NY: Springer Publishing.

Gray, R. H. (1980). *Manual for the provision of intrauterine devices* (p. 98). Geneva, Switzerland: World Health Organization.

Rhoads, J. (2006). *Advanced health assessment and diagnostic reasoning* (p. 341). Philadelphia, PA: Lippincott Williams & Wilkins.

6

The Rectal Exam

R. Mimi Secor

Increasing awareness of anorectal cancer risk and associated risk factors requires heightened vigilance when conducting the rectal exam. Approximately 90% of anal cancers are associated with high-risk human papillomavirus (hr-HPV) infection. Risk factors and risk populations for anal dysplasia include HIV infection; men who have sex with men (MSM); certain immunocompromised conditions such as in transplant patients; history of human papillomavirus (HPV) infection, including anal and/or perineal condyloma; and a history of significant abnormal Papanicolaou (Pap) smears, such as moderate to severe dysplasia, including cervical intraepithelial neoplasia (CIN) 2 and 3, and unprotected anal intercourse.

In this chapter, you will learn:

- The indications for performing a rectal exam
- The technique for performing a rectal examination
- The risk factors and high-risk populations for anal dysplasia
- The technique for performing an anal Pap smear
- How to perform a guaiac stool test for occult blood

THE RECTOVAGINAL EXAM

Considerations for performing a rectovaginal exam include the woman's age (especially older than 50 years); risk factors; and need to more fully assess the uterus, ovaries, rectovaginal septum, and rectum. The rectovaginal exam is particularly helpful if the uterus is retroverted and/or if the ovaries are not palpable vaginally. Other indications include gastrointestinal (GI) complaints, risk factors such as a history of reproductive or GI cancers, an unsatisfactory vaginal bimanual exam, obesity, or when other pathology, such as an ovarian mass, is suspected.

INDICATIONS

The rectal exam may be part of a thorough bimanual exam and should be conducted based on the woman's age, risk factors, medical history, and health status. Generally, a rectal exam is recommended for:

- Women older than 50 years of age
- Younger women based on risk factors and clinical indications

ESSENTIAL FACTS

In certain women, particularly those with a retroverted uterus, obesity, or risks for reproductive cancers, such as ovarian or uterine cancer, the rectal exam may enhance palpating the uterus and ovaries.

The rectal exam may be embarrassing and slightly uncomfortable, but can provide valuable clinical information. It must be performed gently and thoroughly while providing education and emotional support to the woman throughout the exam.

She may be positioned in a supine, lithotomy position utilizing gynaecologic stirrups or in a side-lying position with one or both knees slightly bent.

EXTERNAL RECTAL EXAM

Begin the rectal exam by visually inspecting the external rectal area, using care in separating and inspecting the skin folds that comprise the external sphincter. Note abnormalities, including erythema, whitening, swelling, tenderness, and masses, and other lesions such as fissures, blisters, and ulcers. Next, palpate these tissues and any masses for tenderness, and other abnormal findings.

RECTOVAGINAL EXAM

To prepare for the exam, change gloves and use sufficient lubricant to facilitate the exam and minimize discomfort. Insert your index finger vaginally and your middle finger rectally. Ask the woman to "bear down, relax, and then slowly inhale and exhale." Slide your fingers into place as she is "bearing down" and exhaling. This exam is considered invasive and somewhat uncomfortable (Carcio & Secor, 2015, p. 73).

- Palpate the rectovaginal septum.
- With your other hand on the abdomen, push the uterus as posteriorly as possible.
- With the internal fingers, assess the posterior surface of the uterus and the rectal wall to assess the rectal walls, the rectovaginal septum, and the cul-de-sac for tenderness or masses.
- Note any masses, tenderness, hemorrhoids, or the presence of a retroverted uterus.
- If the uterus is retroverted or retroflexed, the fundus may not be palpable. If palpable, note characteristics such as size, contour, firmness, tenderness, masses, and mobility.
  - If the uterus is retroverted as a result of endometriosis, it may be fixed and nonmobile.
  - Endometriosis may be further evaluated by assessing nodularity of the uterosacral ligaments.

INTERNAL RECTAL EXAM

Perform the internal exam wearing new gloves and using adequate lubrication to facilitate the exam and provide maximum comfort to the woman.

Table 6.1

Assessment Findings of the Rectum and Anus: Normal and Abnormal

Normal	Abnormal
Rectovaginal: areas examined should be smooth, firm, nonfriable, and nontender	Polyps Lesions Hemorrhoids Bleeding following palpation
Palpation of uterus: uncomfortable, but not painful	Pain: suggests endometriosis or PID

PID, pelvic inflammatory disease.

Gently insert one gloved finger and check for unusual tenderness, masses, and any other abnormal findings (Table 6.1). Note the presence, consistency, and color of any stool, and perform a guaiac test to check for occult blood.

Procedure for Guaiac Test

- Upon removal from the rectum, test a guaiac stool sample for occult blood by rolling your third gloved finger onto the test card, when indicated.
- Apply three drops of developing solution to the opposite side of the card.
- The test is positive if you note any blue color.

The guaiac test is most accurate when women perform the test at home after following special dietary restrictions. The woman collects three stool samples on separate days and returns the samples to the office or lab for guaiac testing.

ESSENTIAL FACTS

Colonoscopy is the gold standard test for identifying GI pathology such as polyps and precancerous and cancerous lesions.

ANAL CYTOLOGY

With the risk of anal dysplasia on the rise, increasingly, clinicians are performing anal Pap smears in certain high-risk women. Risk factors, high-risk populations for anal dysplasia, and the recommended procedure for performing an anal Pap smear are reviewed in Exhibit 6.1.

Exhibit 6.1

Procedure for Performing an Anal Pap Smear

Indications
There are no national recommendations, but the following high-risk women may be considered for anal dysplasia/carcinoma screening:

- Current candidates: men who have sex with men (MSM) or HIV-infected persons
- Possible candidates: those who are immunocompromised; those with HPV-related disease, especially vulvar intraepithelial neoplasia (VIN); and men and women with perianal genital warts, or human papillomavirus (HPV)
- Other possible candidates and risk factors: those who have had 15 or more sexual partners, unprotected receptive anal intercourse, a history of cervical intraepithelial neoplasia (CIN), or cigarette smokers

Procedure

- Woman should avoid anal intercourse and douching 24 hours before test.
- Set up supplies and equipment in advance.
- Educate the woman about the procedure and rationale for the test.
- Position her side lying (left side) or in a lithotomy position using gynaecologic stirrups.
- Drape the woman.
- Moisten a Dacron swab with tap water.
  - A cytobrush may be used but can be associated with discomfort.
- Insert the swab or cytobrush approximately 5 cm (2 inches) until the swab reaches the rectal vault.
  - A slight decrease in resistance can be felt.
  - If significant resistance is encountered, remove the swab and redirect the angle or position of the swab.
- Rotate swab 360 degrees.
  - Use a spiral motion and firm pressure against the lateral walls of the anal canal.
  - Circle in one direction only, as reversing direction may remove sample that has been collected.
  - Gradually withdraw over 10 seconds, while still rotating.

(continued)

Exhibit 6.1

Procedure for Performing an Anal Pap Smear (*continued*)

- Agitate sample in liquid fixative for 10 to 15 seconds.
- Label sample as "anal source."

Interpretation of Results

- Anal Pap smears are interpreted using similar nomenclature and classifications as cervical Pap smears: negative for malignancy, atypical squamous cells of unclear significance (ASC-US), suspect high-grade lesion (ASC-H), low-grade squamous intraepithelial lesion (LSIL), high-grade squamous intraepithelial lesion (HSIL).
- No reflex HPV testing is currently available.
- Anal abnormalities are referred for high-resolution anoscopy (HRA) and possible biopsy.

ESSENTIAL FACTS

Sample Documentation of a Complete Gynaecologic Exam With Normal Findings

External genitalia: Normal distribution of pubic hair and normal anatomy; no masses, lesions, abnormal discharge, or tenderness

Vagina: Pink; rugated without bulging or lesions; scant, opaque white discharge without odor; good muscle tone; vaginal pH 4.0 to 4.6 (normal), amine/KOH (potassium hydroxide) test negative, vaginal microscopy negative for clue cells, trichomonads, yeast forms, or white blood cells (WBCs)

Cervix: Pink, smooth, no lesions or mucopus; nontender, no cervical motion tenderness (CMT)

Uterus: Anteverted; normal size, shape, contour (NSSC); mobile; nontender; without palpable masses

Adnexae: Ovaries palpated, normal size, nontender, and no masses palpated

Rectovaginal: No lesions, masses, or fissures; nontender; small amount of brown, soft stool present; guaiac test negative

Reference

Carcio, H. A., & Secor, M. C. (2015). *Advanced health assessment of women: Clinical skills and procedures* (2nd ed.). New York, NY: Springer Publishing.

II

Approach to Examining Special Populations

Many factors can contribute to challenging pelvic exams. Some challenges occur related to the normal aging process, such as menopause-associated vulvovaginal atrophy, and others are related to specific events, such as previous assault and trauma. Depending on age, body type, and childbirth history, normal pelvic landmarks may shift and certain pelvic structures can be difficult to locate. In this part of the book, we provide practical suggestions for the resolution of some of the more common difficulties you may encounter in practice.

7

Specific "Challenges"

Heidi Collins Fantasia

The ability to adequately visualize both the external and internal genitalia is foundational to performing a complete pelvic exam. Many factors can interfere with the clinician's ability to see and examine pelvic organs. This chapter reviews important steps that can help the clinician "find" the cervix in challenging clinical situations and improve comfort for women who are experiencing pain and vulvar itching.

In this chapter, you will learn:

- Common reasons for difficulty visualizing the cervix
- Recommended strategies for improving visualization
- Tips for increasing comfort during the pelvic exam in women with vulvar pain and itching

DIFFICULT VISUALIZATION OF THE CERVIX

Visualizing the cervix is important to ensure adequate cytology sampling and to assess for any abnormal cervical findings. Even if the clinician is not performing Papanicolaou (Pap) smear testing, the clinician should inspect the cervix for abnormalities such as inflammation, discharge, bleeding, and lesions. The cervix often comes into view after the speculum has been inserted and opened. Occasionally, the cervix may be difficult to view and its visualization may require employing various creative techniques.

A cervix that is not positioned in the midline is difficult to visualize. If you cannot see the cervix easily, withdraw the speculum and manually palpate the cervix to determine its location. Upon reinsertion, the speculum should be angled toward the location where the clinician palpated the cervix. Moving the speculum from side to side slightly and opening it wider may help the cervix come into view.

In addition to repositioning the speculum, repositioning the woman may also be helpful. Instruct her to move down as close to the edge of the table as possible and have her tilt up her hips and buttocks. If she is unable to tilt up her hips sufficiently, placing a small rolled towel under her hips or buttocks may be helpful. You may also ask her to bear down or cough forcefully to bring the cervix into view.

It may also be difficult to visualize a cervix that is located in an extreme posterior position. In that case, palpating the cervix prior to inserting the speculum will usually reveal the posterior location. A standard, disposable plastic speculum may not provide adequate visualization of a cervix in this position, so a large, extra-long speculum may be necessary to complete the exam. Having the woman bear down, flex her hips upward, and retract her knees closer to her body will usually help move the cervix down and forward.

Another reason for not locating the cervix is that the woman has relaxed or weakened vaginal walls that impede visualization. In these situations, excess loose tissue on the lateral walls of the vagina collapse inward and visually obstruct the cervix. You can use a large speculum and open it as wide as possible in order to separate the vaginal walls, or cut the finger off a glove (or use a condom and remove the tip to form an improvised sheath) and place this over the speculum blades to help hold back the vaginal walls once the speculum is opened. A lateral wall retractor can also be used, but is often not commonly available in outpatient settings.

ESSENTIAL FACTS

Documentation

- Document any variations on normal position of pelvic organs. Examples:
  - Cervix is posterior, deviated to the patient's right.
  - Cervix difficult to visualize due to redundant vaginal wall tissue.

Communication

When pelvic exams take extra time or manipulation of equipment and positions, it is not uncommon for women to feel as if there is something wrong with their anatomy that is making it difficult for the clinician to complete the exam. The clinician should reassure the woman, explaining that the cervix, uterus, and ovaries can be in different positions, and this does not necessarily indicate an abnormality. Pregnancy, childbirth, a large weight gain or loss, and menopause can all cause a slight shift in pelvic organs. To decrease anxiety, explain every step and why it is being carried out. Statements such as "I need to move the speculum so I can see your cervix clearly" keep her informed about the exam without suggesting that her body is abnormal.

Follow-Up

Using a few creative techniques, the challenging cervix may be visualized. If a clear view of the cervix is still blocked, the practitioner can attempt a blind sweep of the cervix to obtain a Pap smear specimen. If necessary, the woman can reschedule and the pelvic exam can then be reattempted.

ESSENTIAL FACTS

Repositioning the woman and/or the speculum may bring the cervix into view.

VULVAR AND VAGINAL PAIN

Women who experience pain of the vulvar and vaginal area often have difficulty tolerating the pelvic exam, and clinicians who treat these women need to conduct the exam slowly and gently. Pain can result from trauma or injury to the area, infections, skin conditions such as lichen sclerosis or psoriasis, and thin, dry skin that can occur with menopause. Vulvar pain can also result from vulvodynia, which causes pain, burning, and/or irritation of the vulvar tissues. There is no definitive test for vulvodynia and it is often a diagnosis of exclusion based on her symptoms, presence of allodynia, and lack of any identifiable cause of the pain.

Performing a pelvic exam on a woman with vulvar and/or vaginal pain can be extremely challenging. Using a small or pediatric speculum may help decrease discomfort and allow the clinician to visualize the cervix. If even the smallest speculum causes too much pain, Pap smear collection can be attempted without visualizing the cervix, although it is unlikely that this will result in a sample that includes endocervical cells. Vaginal samples for wet mount examination can be gathered with a swab (see Appendices B and C).

ESSENTIAL FACTS

Documentation
- For women complaining of vulvar and vaginal pain, you must document the location and quality of pain. Examples:
  - Tenderness and allodynia bilaterally with gentle palpation with a cotton swab.
  - Vaginal atrophy and dryness (positive sticky glove test) present from 5 to 7 o'clock at the introitus; able to complete exam with narrow speculum.

Communication

Pain is subjective and therefore the woman will be the best source of information to determine its onset, duration, location, and quality. Also, the clinician should assess any treatments that have been tried and whether they were successful. Women with chronic pain who do not have any outward symptoms often feel as if no one believes their discomfort is real, especially if they have seen many providers for the same issue. It is important to validate her experience, even if a cause cannot be readily identified.

Follow-Up

Follow-up appointments may be offered based on the diagnosis and the severity of the problem to assess response to treatment. Infections, skin conditions, and atrophy can be treated and the internal exam deferred until her symptoms have improved.

VULVAR AND VAGINAL ITCHING

Significant vulvar and vaginal itching can also cause considerable discomfort. Vulvitis can be caused by allergic and contact reactions; inflammatory responses; dermatological conditions; and fungal, viral, and bacterial infections. It is a common gynaecological complaint and results in approximately 17 million office visits each year. Inflammation associated with the underlying cause of the itching makes the skin fragile, and often women with vulvar itching will have excoriated skin from scratching and inflammation. It is not uncommon to see fissuring and cracking of the genital skin, especially if the itching and/or condition is chronic (Table 7.1).

Inspection of the genital skin shows the extent of erythema, irritation, or excoriation associated with inflammation and itching. Skin is often tender and sensitive to touch. Clinicians should be gentle and take care not to injure the skin further during the exam. If the condition is acute and the woman is due for a routine exam with Pap smear, it may be advisable to treat the immediate problem and reschedule the routine exam after healing has occurred. Swabs for wet mount examination can be taken without the use of a speculum, and testing for gonorrhea and chlamydia can be done with a urine or vaginal sample.

Table 7.1

Common Causes of Vulvar Itching and Associated Treatment

Possible causes	Treatment
Fungal infections (yeast)	Topical and oral antifungal medications
Bacterial infections (BV)	Oral and topical antibiotics
Sexually transmitted infections	Antibiotics or antivirals specific to the infection
Allergic reactions and/or contact dermatitis	Removal of allergen; topical or oral steroids; antihistamines; sitz baths, improved hygiene, emollients
Skin conditions (lichen simplex chronicus, lichen sclerosus, lichen planus, psoriasis)	Topical steroids, improved hygiene, emollients
Atrophic vaginitis	Local estrogen, improved hygiene, emollients

BV, bacterial vaginosis.

ESSENTIAL FACTS

Documentation
- Areas of redness or excoriation should be documented clearly. Examples:
  - Erythema and fissuring of vulvar bilaterally.
  - Erythema of vaginal walls and introitus especially between 5 and 7 o'clock.
- Any vaginal discharge needs to be noted. Examples:
  - Moderate thin, white discharge coating vaginal walls.
  - Thick, clumpy white discharge present.

Communication

In all cases of vulvar and vaginal itching, an in-office wet prep (wet mount, vaginal microscopy) should be performed to assess for yeast, bacterial vaginosis (BV), trichomoniasis (see Chapter 3), and atrophic vaginitis. Results of the wet prep can be communicated immediately and a treatment plan promptly initiated. Discussions with women need to include education regarding the type of infection and course of treatment. All women with complaints of vulvar and vaginal itching should be discouraged from douching or using strong or drying soaps or scented vaginal hygiene products; wearing tight and restrictive pants and undergarments, especially thong underwear; and shaving pubic hair.

Follow-Up

As with pain, follow-up for vulvar itching will be determined primarily by the diagnosis and choice of treatment. Uncomplicated fungal infections usually respond well to antifungal medications and often clear quickly with treatment. Inflammatory allergic reactions resolve with removal of the allergen. Skin that is extremely excoriated should be reevaluated for healing and monitored for the development of a secondary bacterial infection. A full exam can be deferred until healing is underway and the woman is more comfortable.

ESSENTIAL FACTS

- For women with pain, use the smallest speculum size possible.
- You can gather specimens with a small swab or urine if the woman is unable to tolerate a speculum exam.

For further information related to specific pelvic exam challenges and potential resolutions, please see Appendix A.

8

Examining the Woman With Anxiety, History of Sexual Violence, or Intimate Partner Violence

Heidi Collins Fantasia

Many women are anxious during gynaecologic exams, but some women are extremely anxious. Sometimes a cause for the anxiety cannot be determined, but extreme anxiety can also be associated with specific events, such as a history of physical or sexual abuse. Vaginismus, or abnormal involuntary spasms of the vagina, can be a result of sexual abuse or trauma and causes increased pain and inability to tolerate a gynaecologic exam. During the interviewing process, a thorough psychological, social, family, and sexual history should be obtained, noting evidence of or past history of anxiety, sexual abuse, violence, family trauma, negative gynaecologic experiences, and other factors that might indicate the woman may have difficulty with gynaecologic exams.

In this chapter, you will learn how to:

- Recognize behaviors that signal extreme anxiety and apply strategies to help the woman work through the pelvic exam
- Approach a pelvic exam with a woman who has a history of physical and/or sexual abuse

ANXIETY

A severely anxious woman can be very challenging to examine and make completing a pelvic exam difficult. If the woman has previously had a gynaecologic exam, she should be asked about prior experiences and any difficulties she had. Women who are having their first exam should be told exactly what to expect. They may benefit from seeing the speculum, and some women may want to hold it and try opening and closing it.

Women who are extremely anxious should be talked through the entire exam so they know exactly what is happening and in what order the exam will proceed. Women should know they can ask the clinician to stop the exam at any time and that the clinician will honor the request. Proceed with the exam slowly and gently, communicating in a relaxed and unhurried manner. If the woman is known to the practice and previous exams have been difficult, allow extra time and adjust the schedule to accommodate a longer time slot for this appointment.

Encourage relaxation techniques, including deep breathing, meditation, and imagery. The woman may benefit from the presence of a support person of her choice, and, if possible, should be allowed to have this person present with her for the exam. If speculum insertion is difficult, consider asking her to bear down and breathe deeply. It may take multiple attempts to insert the speculum and complete the exam *over multiple visits and sometimes many months*. Palpating the cervix in advance of the speculum exam may help both the woman and the clinician. Conducting the exam patiently and allowing the woman to control the pace and content of the exam is critical to decreasing anxiety. A woman who senses that the clinician is frustrated and attempting to hurry will probably not be able to relax.

Consider short-acting antianxiety medications in a single dose with no refills if the woman has a support person who is able to drive her home after the exam. The decision to prescribe antianxiety medications should be based on her clinical history, current medications, and preferences. Practitioners should always prescribe the lowest dose possible and inform the woman that the goal is to lessen anxiety, not to eliminate it entirely. Caution should be used in women with a history of substance abuse or avoided completely if there are concerns about sobriety and/or relapse. All antianxiety medications have side effects

Table 8.1

Short-Acting Antianxiety Medications (Benzodiazepines)[a]

Medication (generic and brand names)	Single dose (mg) prior to exam
Lorazapam (Ativan)	0.5, 1, or 2
Alprazolam (Xanax)	0.25, 0.5, 1, or 2
Clonazepam (Klonopin)	0.5, 1, or 2
Diazepam (Valium)	2, 5, or 10

[a]These medications should be used with caution, especially with women who have a history of addiction, who are taking other central nervous system (CNS) depressants, or have a current or previous history of mental health issues.

of drowsiness and dizziness and women should be informed of this. See Table 8.1 for common antianxiety medications and available doses. It is often helpful to have women take the prescribed dose 30 minutes prior to the exam.

ESSENTIAL FACTS

Documentation

- Physiologic signs of anxiety should be documented. Examples:
  - Tachycardic, HR 94.
  - Patient diaphoretic, tense, and guarding.
- The extent to which the exam can be completed is documented. Examples:
  - Exam performed; bimanual limited by *patient anxiety, unable to accurately assess uterus and ovaries*.
  - Unable to insert speculum or perform bimanual exam *due to anxiety and/or pain when exam attempted*.

Communication

Women with extreme anxiety are often upset over the difficulties with the exam and apologetic that the process takes longer than usual or is incomplete. Clinicians should remain patient, calm, and understanding, as their anxiety or frustration will only increase the woman's anxiety. Each aspect of the exam should be done slowly, at a pace that is set by the woman. It is important for the clinician to communicate what is happening during each step. This will allow the woman to decide whether she is able to continue. At the completion of the exam, the woman should be informed of all findings and whether any follow-up is needed.

Follow-Up

If the exam can be completed *and is normal,* then follow-up is not necessary. If anxiety prevents all or part of the exam, then a plan should be made for repeating the exam at a different time. If this is necessary, strategies can be implemented to address the woman's anxiety and therefore increase the likelihood the next exam will be successful. If anxiety is extreme, referral to a therapist may help the woman work through underlying issues related to the gynaecologic exam. Bringing a friend and implementing meditation, biofeedback, and other relaxation techniques can also be very effective in reducing anxiety. If anxiety is not specific to the gynaecologic exam and is part of an overall anxiety disorder, referral to a mental health provider should be considered to have mental health issues evaluated and treated.

ESSENTIAL FACTS

- Encourage use of a mirror and the woman's involvement during the exam process.
- Proceed with the exam slowly and thoroughly, and explain the exam simply (especially in advance) to decrease anxiety.
- Encourage relaxation techniques and deep breathing.
- Consider short-acting antianxiety medications in a single dose if appropriate for the woman and situation.

PHYSICAL AND SEXUAL VIOLENCE

Performing a pelvic exam on a woman with a history of physical/sexual abuse can be especially challenging. It is extremely important not to revictimize the woman during the exam. Exposure and touching the pelvic area and positioning for the exam often bring up memories of the abuse. Many women who have experienced sexual abuse or assault do not disclose this to their health care providers. Researchers who conducted the National Intimate Partner and Sexual Violence Survey reported that approximately one third of women in the United States have experienced intimate partner violence (IPV) at some point in their lifetime and nearly half have experienced sexual violence (Black et al., 2011).

Victims of sexual violence may demonstrate certain behaviors that suggest a history of abuse. During an examination, the woman may be reluctant to undress and allow the clinician access to her pelvic and genital area. Women who have been victims of sexual violence may also move away as the clinician attempts to insert the speculum or may close her legs tightly. Arching her back off the exam table and having a rigidly tense posture are also actions that are common for violence victims as are crying, shaking, hiding under the drape sheet, or complete disassociation and separation from the exam.

For women with a known history of sexual abuse or violence, having control over the flow and timing of the exam is crucial. The visit often takes much longer, and an exam may be impossible or require multiple visits to complete. Violence victims need to feel secure, and therefore the process from introduction and first visit to the completion of a full exam can take many visits or even years as the woman learns to trust the provider and feel safe. Women who have experienced any form of sexual violence should always be greeted and interviewed while fully clothed.

Before beginning any part of the exam, let the woman know exactly what to expect. Some women feel more comfortable if they have a support person with them and the clinician should always try to accommodate this request. Being completely undressed is often difficult for women who have experienced sexual violence. Allowing a woman who has experienced sexual violence to keep on some clothing, such as her shirt, may increase her comfort.

There are other important steps the clinician can take when performing a gynaecologic exam on a woman who has been a victim of sexual violence. Letting the woman set the pace of the exam and have control over certain actions can enhance empowerment and increase the chance of a nontraumatic exam. Women may wish to use a mirror and insert the speculum themselves. The speculum should be warm, the smallest size possible, and inserted slowly. Lubricant should be used to decrease discomfort. Consider alternate positions, such as semireclining without using the stirrups. Assess her anxiety and level of tolerance for the exam multiple times. Let her know that the examination will stop at any point if she is having difficulty completing the exam.

If it is impossible to complete the exam, she may require a step-by-step desensitization process. Over the course of multiple appointments, she can become more familiar with the environment and exam process. At this point, the clinician might consider comanaging care with a counselor who has expertise in working with women who have been affected by sexual violence.

When caring for a woman who has experienced a recent sexual assault or sexual trauma, the genital area should be examined carefully. According to Brown and Muscari (2010), many health care providers use the TEARS pneumonic to describe the different types of genital injuries. Becoming familiar with this pneumonic will assist the clinician in identifying the constellation of injuries that are often experienced by victims of sexual assault:

T = tears, any break in tissue integrity
E = ecchymosis, any discoloration of skin or mucous membranes; also called *bruising*
A = abrasion, skin excoriations caused by the removal of the most superficial layer of skin
R = redness, erythematous skin that is abnormally inflamed because of irritation
S = swelling, edematous, or transient engorgement of tissues

Brown and Muscari also report the "common genital injuries in elder victims of sexual assault are lacerations, abrasions, and bruises" (2010, p. 185).

Sommers (2007) identifies the most common locations for injury as:

- Posterior fourchette
- Labia minora
- Hymen
- Fossa navicularis

However, not all women who report an incident of sexual assault will present with obvious signs of trauma to the genital area. The exam should proceed objectively without any judgment or bias from the clinician.

ESSENTIAL FACTS

Documentation

- With a remote history of sexual assault, documentation includes the woman's emotional response to the exam. Examples:
  - Mild anxiety verbalized but able to tolerate exam without incident.
  - Unable to complete exam due to anxiety and emotional distress.

Communication

The timing of sexual violence will often guide the discussion before and after the exam. Screening all women for a current and past history of physical and sexual violence is essential and supported by major organizations such as the American College of Obstetricians and Gynecologists (ACOG), the American Medical Association (AMA), the Institute of Medicine (IOM), and the American Academy of Pediatrics (AAP). Simple screening questions, such as "Have you ever been forced to have sex when you didn't want to?" will help assist with disclosure and focus of the exam and follow-up. If the physical or sexual violence has occurred in the past and the woman is stable and out of immediate danger, then the conversation will focus on the woman's feelings toward the exam, any previous difficulties she has encountered, and what can be done to increase her comfort with the present exam. If the physical or sexual violence was recent or ongoing and the woman has not received evaluation and health care since the most recent incident, the conversation will be very different. If sexual violence has occurred during the past 5 to 7 days, the woman should be informed about the collection of forensic evidence (see Follow-Up section). If it has been more than 5 to 7 days since the sexual violence, the practitioner should ask about the woman's immediate concerns, such as pregnancy or sexually transmitted infections (STIs).

INTIMATE PARTNER VIOLENCE

Caring for a woman who has experienced physical, psychological, or emotional violence from a current or former intimate partner is similar to the care of women who are victims of sexual violence because often the two forms of violence occur simultaneously. One in three women or approximately 33% of women have experienced physical violence by an intimate partner (Black et al., 2011). Women are often reluctant to disclose IPV and it may take multiple visits before an atmosphere of trust exists and a woman feels comfortable disclosing the violence to a health care provider. Women who have been victims of IPV often have the same difficulties with a pelvic exam as do women who have been victims of sexual abuse. Techniques, such as approaching the exam slowly and allowing the woman to control what happens with her body, will be just as important for women with a history of IPV as for women with a history of sexual violence.

Communication

Nonjudgmental and consistent screening for IPV is the first step to increasing the chances that a woman will disclose a history of violence. Although rates of reporting are low, women are more likely to disclose if asked about violence directly. This can be accomplished through standardized screening questions such as: "Have you ever been abused or felt unsafe in relationship (physical/sexual/emotional threats or violence)?" and "Are you currently afraid of anyone?" These types of screening questions should be incorporated into the standardized patient history and intake forms and reviewed with women at each visit. They can also be grouped with questions about sexual violence so that the most sensitive questions are asked together. Making violence screening a standard protocol ensures that all women, regardless of age, sexual orientation, gender identification, marital status, race, ethnicity, relationship status, and other sociodemographic factors, are screened equally and without bias. It is important to frame questions about physical and sexual violence in a nonjudgmental way and to let women know that questions of this type are asked of everyone so that individual women do not feel threatened or singled out for what has happened to them.

Follow-Up

A woman's ability to tolerate gynaecologic exams after a history of physical or sexual violence will vary widely. Some women may experience only mild anxiety, whereas others will exhibit symptoms of severe distress. Follow-up plans will be based on her symptoms and feelings about the exam. For those with acute distress that prevents completion of a pelvic exam, follow-up and comanagement with a therapist or counselor are often helpful. If the abuse or assault was recent and the clinician is the first provider whom the woman has encountered, he or she should provide information about rape crisis centers and options regarding reporting to law enforcement. If assaulted within the past 5 to 7 days, the woman should be informed that forensic evidence can be collected, although the exact time frame for collection can range from 3 to 7 days and varies from state to state. This is best done by a provider who has specialized experience and training in sexual assault exams and may require the woman to visit a hospital emergency department that is designated as a site that can provide forensic evidence collection. The clinician should be aware of what services are available in his or her practice area if referrals are needed. Additional follow-up for repeat STI or pregnancy testing can also be scheduled based on the timing of the sexual violence.

For women who disclose an experience of ongoing physical violence in a current relationship, the clinician must do a lethality assessment and start a discussion about whether she has the ability to leave the relationship. Many barriers to leaving an abusive relationship exist for women who are experiencing IPV, including social isolation, financial control, and lack of resources for housing, child care, transportation, and legal assistance. Women who are not documented face additional barriers that coexist with their immigration status, including fear of incarceration, deportation, and loss of parental rights. Providers can assist women in starting a safety plan that includes the resources they will need to leave the relationship. It may take women an extended period of time to leave a violent relationship. Clinicians should always have an updated list of local resources, including law enforcement, as well as legal, counseling, and shelter services. If women are unable to immediately terminate a violent relationship, then reassessing safety, plans, and available resources at each visit is essential.

ESSENTIAL FACTS

- Screen for physical and sexual violence at every visit.
- A successful exam may take months or years to complete.
- Consider comanagement with a counselor.
- Use slow, gentle movements and allow the woman to direct the pace of the exam.

HUMAN TRAFFICKING

Human trafficking can be viewed as a subset of sexual violence and abuse. Commercial sexual exploitation is the most common reason for human trafficking, and adolescents and young women are most at risk. Because of the secretive nature of trafficking, it is difficult to accurately determine the scope of the problem, but it is estimated that more than 14,000 young women and girls are trafficked in the United States each year.

It is very hard to determine whether a woman is being trafficked, as often there are no definitive signs and the woman will appear outwardly to be well assimilated into the community. A woman who is being trafficked is under the control of a pimp who is the gatekeeper to her health care access. Therefore, these women often do not receive routine care. Instead, they present for episodic office visits when there is a problem or concern that is usually related to a gynaecologic issue.

The signs of trafficking can be vague and, if they appear individually, may not be enough to raise concern. As with all cases of violence, the woman's stated history of the illness or injury may not match with the exam findings, or there may be inconsistencies in her account of the problem. A male partner's refusal to leave the woman alone in the exam room or a partner who appears impatient about the length of the office visit may also be indications of control and abuse. Other possible signs of human trafficking include multiple pregnancies and pregnancy terminations, STIs, inconsistent and episodic health care, and overt signs of trauma such as bruising, burns, cuts, and a history of bone fractures. Table 8.2 includes a list of possible signs of human trafficking.

Table 8.2

Possible Warning Signs of Human Trafficking

- Homelessness, frequent address changes, inconsistent health care
- Presence of an older boyfriend or age disparity in an intimate or sexual relationship
- Signs of violence and/or psychological trauma (including mental illness and suicide attempts)
- History of criminal behavior or involvement with youth services
- Travel with an older male who is not a guardian
- History of family violence
- Younger than age 18 and involved in or history of prior prostitution

- Chronic runaway (adolescents)
- Unique tattoos (used to mark victim as property of pimp)
- STIs, pregnancy, history of pregnancy terminations
- Substance use/abuse
- Access to material things that the woman/adolescent cannot afford
- History of rape or child sexual abuse
- Not attending school, frequent absences, or academic failures (adolescents)

STIs, sexually transmitted infections.

Source: Adapted from U.S. Department of Health and Human Services (2009).

ESSENTIAL FACTS

Documentation

- Because there are usually no definitive signs of human trafficking, documentation needs to accurately describe both the woman's history and physical exam findings. Examples:
  - Recently relocated to area, states unemployed, last gyn exam >2 years ago.
  - Complaining of pelvic pain, vaginal discharge ×3 weeks.
  - 4-cm yellow bruise on inner aspect of left thigh; pt does not recall injury.

Communication

It is important to establish an open and safe dialogue in all cases of suspected trafficking. Women who are trafficked often fear retaliation from a pimp if the lifestyle is discovered, and they are never sure whom they can trust. Therefore, they are reluctant to disclose a history of abuse. Pimps may threaten with physical harm, deportation if in the country illegally, or harm to family members if the woman divulges the trafficking. Questions for the woman should start with a general health history that includes social aspects, such as work, school, housing, and finances/health insurance. More specific inquiries include questions related to physical and sexual health and safety. Examples of more direct questions are: "Have you been physically or emotionally hurt or threatened by anyone, including a sex partner?" "Have you ever been forced to have sex when you didn't want to?" "Have you ever exchanged sex for drugs, money, food, or a place to live?" and "Have you ever been threatened with harm if you did not perform sexual acts in exchange for money?"

Follow-Up

Scheduling exam follow-ups can also be challenging. Pimps are typically reluctant to bring these women in for even one visit and can become suspicious if it is recommended that the woman be seen again. If a follow-up exam is scheduled, it is not uncommon for the woman to miss the visit and have contact information that is not valid. These women are moved around frequently and often do not stay in one area long enough to establish consistent health care, although they may come back to the practice after a long absence.

All health care providers should be aware of local recourses in their practice area for women who are victims or suspected victims of abuse. As with IPV, those who traffic women use multiple control tactics, including financial control, social isolation, physical control/abuse, and psychological abuse. Leaving a pimp is dangerous and complicated; often these women have no money or personal possessions other than what they are wearing. If the woman is a minor, laws regarding statutory rape and mandatory reporting vary from state to state. All health care providers need to have a list of shelters, abuse hotlines, community advocates, and local law enforcement agencies that can be provided to women.

ESSENTIAL FACTS

- Sexual trafficking is the most common form of human trafficking.
- Signs of human trafficking are often vague and difficult to determine.
- Gynaecologic complaints are common among women who are trafficked.

References

Black, M. C., Basile, K. C., Breiding, M. J., Smith, S. G., Walters, M. L., Merrick, M. T., . . . & Stevens, M. R. (2011). The National Intimate Partner and Sexual Violence Survey (NISVS): 2010 summary report. Atlanta, GA: National Center for Injury Prevention and Control, Centers for Disease Control and Prevention. Retrieved from https://www.cdc.gov/violenceprevention/pdf/nisvs_report2010-a.pdf

Brown, K. M., & Muscari, M. E. (2010). *Quick reference to adult and older adult forensics: A guide for nurses and other health care professionals* (p. 170). New York, NY: Springer Publishing.

Sommers, M. (2007). Defining patterns of genital injury from sexual assault: A review. *Trauma, Violence, & Abuse*, 8(3), 270–280.

U.S. Department of Health and Human Services. (2009). Resources: Common health issues seen in victims of human trafficking. Look beneath the surface: Restore and rescue. Retrieved from https://www.acf.hhs.gov/trafficking/index.html

9

Examining Premenarchal Children, Adolescents, and Virginal Women

Heidi Collins Fantasia

Women who have never been sexually active and premenarchal children do not require the same screening tests as sexually active adolescents or adult women. Often, gynaecologic visits for this group are problem focused, with women seeking care for specific concerns such as vulvar complaints, vaginitis, abnormal vaginal bleeding, or discomfort. Pelvic exams for these women should focus on the specific patient concern and be limited to what the patient is able to tolerate.

In this chapter, you will learn how to:

- Apply alternate approaches to performing a pelvic exam on a child
- Employ strategies for completing a pelvic exam with virginal women
- Recognize situations that warrant specialist referral or delayed/deferred exam

CHILDREN AND PREMENARCHAL PATIENTS

To successfully perform a gynaecologic exam of a young child or a child who has not yet reached menarche, the clinician must approach the exam differently than with an adult. Some special considerations to keep in mind when working with very young children and premenarchal girls include:

- The exam cannot be hurried or rushed, and the clinician must be gentle, patient, and understanding of both the child's and parent's anxiety.
- Schedule extra time for the exam, especially if the child is new to the practice and not familiar with the staff and office.
- Place all instruments out of sight.
- The clinician should consider removing the lab coat.

Obtaining a history from a child can be challenging, especially with very young children. Parents will often provide the majority of the child's health history and the reason for the visit. Even verbal and social children will often be extremely quiet in a new setting when they are nervous and anxious. For some children, pictures or dolls can be helpful tools to determine level of pain or location of a problem. Crying, fussing, and clinging to a parent are all normal childhood responses to fear and discomfort and should be anticipated during the visit.

Tanner Staging

Knowledge of children's growth and development is necessary for any health care providers who work with children. Pubertal changes and maturation occur in a sequential, predictable manner and are visible through the appearance of secondary sex characteristics. The average age for first appearance of pubic hair varies depending on race and ethnicity, but typically ranges from 9 to 10 years of age.

The staging system for pubertal development that is most commonly used is referred to as *Tanner stages* (Figure 9.1). For females, these stages describe breast and pubic hair development, but for the purposes of this chapter the focus will be on pubic hair changes only. The stages range from 1 to 5, with 1 representing a preadolescent with no pubic hair and 5 representing the pubic hair pattern of an adult woman.

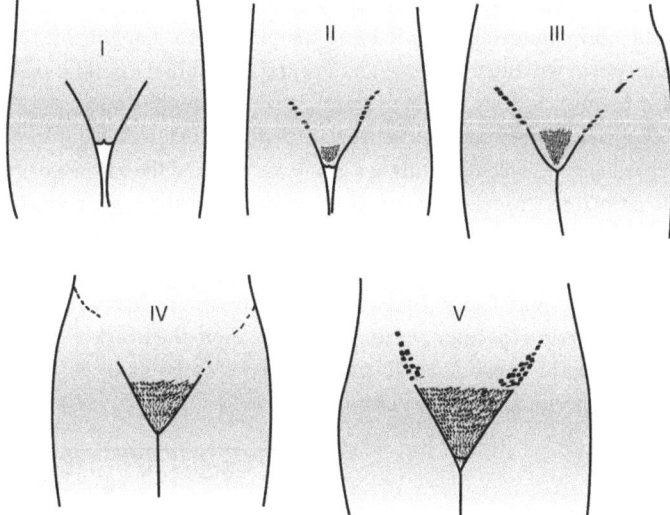

Figure 9.1 Tanner stages of pubic hair development.

Tanner Stages of Pubic Hair in Girls

Stage 1: Prepubertal (velus hair similar to abdominal wall)
Stage 2: Sparse growth of long, slightly pigmented hair, straight or curled, along labia
Stage 3: Darker, coarser, and curlier hair, spreading sparsely over pubic area
Stage 4: Adult-type hair, covering smaller area with no spread to medial surface of thighs
Stage 5: Hair is adult-like in type and quantity, with horizontal distribution (adapted from www.ncbi.nlm.nih.gov/books/NBK138588)

Examining Children

Emphasize that the majority of the exam will be "just looking," without having to touch. Use of stirrups will be determined based on age, understanding, and anxiety level of the child. Older children will most likely be able to tolerate positioning with stirrups. For young children, alternate positions are best. The child can remain on the parent's lap in a frog-legged position, or this position can also be used on an exam table if the child does not fit comfortably in the parent's lap. A lateral side-lying position is also an option if this makes the child more comfortable. Undressing completely and changing into an exam gown will often increase anxiety and therefore the child should only remove clothing that is necessary to complete the exam.

Gynaecologic exams on children are primarily external. Significant gynaecologic problems in this age group are rare and the vast majority of complaints are related to vulvovaginitis. Often the vagina can be visualized by asking the child to cough or bear down. Any specimens can be collected from the vaginal introitus with a small swab without using a speculum. Older children who are closer to menarche may be able to tolerate a speculum exam. In this situation, the smallest speculum should be used. A nasal otoscope may also be used when the smallest speculum is still too large.

ESSENTIAL FACTS

Documentation
- Documentation should include reference to positioning during the exam. Examples:
    - Patient examined frog-legged on exam table, supported by mother.
- Information should be provided about exam findings. Examples:
    - External vulvar erythema of the labia minora and majora, present bilaterally.
    - No evidence of foreign body at introitus with coughing.

Communication

When performing an exam on a child, the clinician's communication will alternate between the child and the parent. If the child is a toddler with limited language, the majority of the history and symptoms will be elicited from the parent. Although the clinician can obtain a large portion of the history from the parents, children can help give concrete facts about symptoms and their location, especially if they are school aged or older. Ask short, direct questions using language that the child will understand. Parents can provide you with terms they use for different body parts and bodily functions. When talking, the clinician should be sitting at eye level with the child and allow adequate time for the child to give her answer.

Follow-Up

If necessary, plans for follow-up care should be made after a discussion of exam findings with the child's parents. If a speculum exam is necessary because pathology or a foreign body is suspected, the clinician should consider a referral to a pediatric gynaecologist, especially for very young children. Exams of this nature may need to be conducted under anesthesia or ultrasound guidance. In cases of suspected child sexual abuse, referrals should be initiated for a sexual assault forensic exam and local child services and law enforcement agencies must be notified.

ESSENTIAL FACTS

- Gynaecologic exams on children consist primarily of inspection of the external genitalia and most do not require a speculum.
- If a more detailed internal exam is necessary, referral to a pediatric gynaecologist should be considered.
- If the history reveals possible sexual abuse of a child, immediate referral to a pediatric sexual assault nurse examiner is recommended.

For additional information related to specific pelvic exam challenges and potential resolutions, please see Appendix A.

ADOLESCENTS

Adolescence is the longest developmental stage, often seen as beginning with the onset of puberty and extending through the college years into the early to mid-20s. It can be viewed as the period between sexual maturation and the attainment of adult roles and responsibilities. Characterized by rapid physical growth, reproductive maturity, and psychosocial expectations, adolescence is often the most tumultuous developmental stage to navigate.

Clinicians who work with adolescent women must understand brain development and its impact on behavior. Significant brain development in adolescence occurs in neurologic regions and systems that play a pivotal role, not only in regulation of behavior, emotion, and sensation, but also in the perception and evaluation of risk and reward. This can result in decisions that put adolescents at risk for injury because of their inability to recognize the risk and potential harm associated with various behaviors.

Examining Adolescents

Clinicians must approach the adolescent pelvic exam with patience. Although adolescents often have the physical appearance of an adult, emotional development varies widely and adolescent women can be apprehensive, nervous, and embarrassed to discuss sexual topics and have their genital area examined. The scope of the adolescent gynaecologic visit will differ depending on the individual reason for seeking health care. For example, if the visit is to begin or maintain contraception, no pelvic exam is required (except in the case of insertion of an intrauterine device [IUD]). If the adolescent is complaining of a specific problem, such as a bleeding abnormality, pelvic pain, or vaginal discharge, then speculum and/or bimanual exam will be required in order to establish a diagnosis and treatment plan. Breast exams are not recommended for adolescent women who do not present with breast complaints and therefore most adolescents need only undress from the waist down to complete the pelvic exam. For contraceptive visits, there is no reason to change into an examination robe and the appointment can be completed without undressing.

ESSENTIAL FACTS

Documentation
- Documentation should include a reference to the reason for the visit. Examples:
  - Patient requesting start of oral contraception, denies any gynaecologic complains.
  - Patient complaining of increased vaginal discharge and postcoital spotting.
- Information should be provided about exam findings. Examples:
  - Breast and pelvic exam deferred. No contraindications to combined oral contraception.
  - Cervix friable with copious yellow discharge. Gonorrhea and chlamydia testing done.

Communication

Adolescents should be the primary source of information, although a parent or guardian may provide additional details about family or childhood history that the adolescent is unable to remember. If an adolescent woman is accompanied by a parent or guardian, the clinician should elicit a confidential sexual history with just the adolescent present so the young woman can answer questions honestly, especially if there is information she prefers not to share with a parent. This also helps to establish trust between the clinician and the adolescent. However, clinicians should be clear regarding what information can be kept confidential. If the adolescent discloses thoughts or actions of harm to either herself or others, a serious or life-threatening condition is discovered, or evidence of sexual or physical abuse is present, then confidentiality cannot be guaranteed.

In addition to addressing the adolescent woman's reason for seeking care, this visit allows the clinician an opportunity to provide education and anticipatory guidance. Even if the adolescent is not sexually active, a discussion about sexually transmitted infections (STIs) and pregnancy should take place. Plans for future sexual activity should be assessed and anticipatory information provided on the prevention of infections and unintended pregnancy. Preventative counseling on risk factors, such as smoking, alcohol and drug use, and the dangers of driving while impaired or riding in a car with an impaired driver needs to be completed in a clear and nonjudgmental manner.

Follow-Up

Timing and scope of follow-up appointments will depend on the reason for the visit. Initial contraceptive prescriptions usually have follow-up within the first 3 months after initiation, but exact timing will vary depending on the specific method. A focused problem may not necessarily require a subsequent visit. An uncomplicated yeast vaginitis that responds to treatment does not warrant follow-up, however pelvic pain and menstrual irregularities should be investigated after treatment or diagnostic studies.

ESSENTIAL FACTS

- Clinicians need to have a thorough understanding of adolescent growth and development.
- Adolescent women should be interviewed privately without parents or guardians present.
- Reason for visit will determine scope of exam.

10

Useful Techniques When Examining Overweight, Multiparous, or Physically Challenged Women

Heidi Collins Fantasia

Examining women who are obese, multiparous, or who have physical conditions that limit their mobility can be very challenging for both the clinician and the woman. Often, adjustments need to be made to the physical office space and equipment. Preparing for the exam in advance, and allowing extra time for the exam, will increase the woman's comfort and chances for a successful exam. In addition, extra staff may be needed to assist with transfers, positioning, safety, and specimen collection.

In this chapter, you will learn how to:

- Identify specific challenges to performing a pelvic exam on women who are obese
- Identify physical changes that are common with multiparity
- List strategies to accommodate women who are physically challenged

OBESITY

Obese women are less likely to receive routine gynaecologic care than are women with a body mass index (BMI) in the healthy or normal range. Weight bias and fear of judgment may contribute to avoidance of gynaecologic care. Exam tables, equipment, and gowns are often inadequate, especially for morbidly obese women. The clinician needs to be sensitive to the needs of overweight and obese women and adjust his or her exam techniques accordingly.

Impaired mobility may be the first challenge when working with obese patients. Often, positioning on the exam table can be difficult. Exam tables are narrow and women who are obese or morbidly obese may feel as if they will fall off. Once on the table, obese women may have less ability to flex and rotate their hips when positioning in the stirrups.

Clinicians may need staff assistance when performing the pelvic exam. Employing a few helpful techniques serves to reduce or avoid embarrassment for the obese woman who has presented for care. These include the following:

- The woman's thighs may need to be retracted when in the stirrups. An assistant can help gently hold back any skin folds that are obscuring the vulva and vagina.
- Obese women often have excess vaginal skin and tissue that can make visualizing the cervix challenging. Using a larger speculum and palpating the cervix prior to inserting the speculum will help facilitate the exam.
- Asking the woman to flex her hips upward may also bring the cervix into a better position for viewing.
- Once the speculum is inserted and opened, it may still be difficult to visualize the cervix. Speculums lack lateral support, and thus the vaginal sidewalls can collapse inward and obscure the view of the cervix. This is especially true if using a disposable, plastic speculum. In this situation, cutting off the closed end of a condom or glove finger and slipping this over the closed blades of a metal speculum is very helpful. When opened, the sheath assists in holding back any redundant tissue that may block the cervix.

Bimanual exams are often less sensitive due to excess adipose tissue, especially if the woman has a large abdominal pannus. If the clinician is having difficulty palpating through extra lower abdominal tissue, the woman may be able to help by holding back the skin in this area. If the clinician is unable to adequately assess the uterus and ovaries and the woman and/or the clinician suspect pathology, ultrasound evaluation of the pelvic organs may be a useful option.

ESSENTIAL FACTS

Documentation

- Any difficulty with the exam or inability to adequately assess internal organs should be documented. Examples:
  - Exam limited by abdominal obesity.
  - Unable to assess uterus and ovaries due to body habitus and/or abdominal obesity.

Communication

Obese and overweight women often face societal discrimination because of their body size. Many avoid routine health care because of anxiety over being weighed and fear of judgment by health care providers. Statements such as "You need to lose weight" or "Your BMI is too high" are unhelpful and often frustrating. Care should be taken to discuss weight-related issues in terms of concern over actual or potential health consequences. Framing this topic as part of overall health promotion will assist women in hearing a message of concern rather than a lecture about the health consequences of obesity.

Statements that show understanding and concern regarding specific complaints are far more effective than general declarations about obesity. For example, stating, "Heavy menstrual periods can be one complication of obesity. Reducing your weight will often help reduce bleeding. Let's talk about a plan to set weight-loss goals and monitor your menstrual cycles," shows that the clinician understands the significance of the problem and the clinician cares about finding a solution. It is far more effective than saying, "You need to lose weight to help decrease the bleeding." In addition, some women are not ready to make the necessary diet and lifestyle changes that will result in weight loss. Asking questions such as, "Have you thought about losing weight?" or "Do you want to lose weight?" will allow the provider to understand the woman's goals and provide context for discussions.

If the exam is limited by obesity, the woman should be told in a clear, nonjudgmental manner. Women have a right and responsibility to understand the findings of the health care visit. "Because of the shape and size of your body, I wasn't able to feel your uterus and ovaries" is a direct and factual statement about the limitations of the exam. This will allow for discussion about whether further evaluation is necessary.

Follow-Up

A decision to recommend additional evaluation of the obese woman will depend on presenting symptoms and exam findings. In the presence of normal menstrual cycles and no gynaecologic-related complaints, a limited exam may not require any follow-up other than reevaluation at the next scheduled health care visit. If the woman presents with complaints of menstrual irregularities, pain, or other symptoms that suggest a gynaecologic origin, then additional evaluation is warranted. Most often this can be accomplished with pelvic ultrasound.

ESSENTIAL FACTS

- Using a wider, larger speculum may help bring the cervix into view.
- Palpating the cervix prior to inserting the speculum will assist with location.
- Asking the woman to flex/lift up her hips can change the position of the cervix.
- Placing a condom or finger of a glove with one end cut off over a metal speculum can hold back the lateral walls of the vagina and allow the cervix to be seen.
- Placing a towel or small pillow under the woman's hips may also help the clinician visualize the cervix.

MULTIPARITY

The main challenges associated with multiparity are related to lax muscles in the vaginal wall or pelvic floor. Childbirth and multiple deliveries can weaken pelvic muscles and contribute to uterine prolapse, cystocele, and rectocele formation. When these conditions occur, it is often difficult to locate the cervix because landmarks can change and bulging in the vaginal walls may block visualization of the cervix. In addition, after pregnancy and delivery, the cervix may move to a posterior position, which can make it more difficult to see with an average-sized speculum.

Locating/palpating the cervix manually prior to speculum insertion will help identify its position and assist in determining whether the cervix is located posteriorly. Some helpful techniques include the following:

- If the cervix appears to be posterior, use a longer speculum for adequate visualization and specimen collection.
- If weakened vaginal muscles or bulging from the bladder or rectum obscures the cervix, proceed as with obese women.
- Reposition the woman so her hips tilt upward and place a sheath over the speculum blades to hold back any tissue that is blocking the cervix.

ESSENTIAL FACTS

Documentation

- It is important to document the location of pelvic anatomy. Examples:
  - Parous os, posterior. Cervix visualized with long speculum.
  - Mild uterine prolapse, cervix located at midvagina.
  - Moderate uterine prolapse, cervix at vaginal introitus.

Communication

Multiparous women should have the findings of their exam communicated in a straightforward manner, using correct anatomical terms for anatomy and physical findings. Care should be taken to avoid suggesting that childbirth has "stretched out" the vagina or caused their uterus, bladder, or rectum to "fall." Women should be reassured that pregnancy and delivery may change the shape and location of the cervix, but that this is a normal and expected finding that does not need any intervention. The presence of a cystocele, rectocele, or uterine prolapse should be discussed in terms of possible symptoms, side effects, and whether the degree of organ prolapse requires further evaluation and intervention.

Follow-Up

Further evaluation is determined by the severity of any abnormal findings and whether the woman is experiencing discomfort or adverse effects. There are many options to strengthen pelvic floor muscle tone. Women can be taught to perform Kegel exercises by contracting (squeezing) the muscles normally used to stop urine flow. Muscles should be contracted for a few seconds and then released. This is repeated 10 to 15 times. This cycle of contracting and releasing the pelvic floor muscles should be done at least three times throughout the day. Also, women can be referred to physical therapy to specifically target the pelvic floor. Surgical evaluation should be considered if the uterus is prolapsed to the vaginal introitus or beyond, or if urinary and fecal incontinence is significantly decreasing the woman's quality of life and interfering with daily activities.

ESSENTIAL FACTS

- Palpating the cervix prior to inserting the speculum will assist with location.
- Placing a condom or finger of a glove with one end cut off over a metal speculum can hold back the lateral walls of the vagina and allow the clinician to visualize the cervix.
- Using a wider, longer speculum may help bring the cervix into view.

PHYSICALLY CHALLENGED WOMEN

Women who are disabled or physically challenged face multiple obstacles when accessing health care. This population has the same gynaecologic health care needs as all women; they need access to timely gynaecologic and breast exams in addition to their special health care needs. However, chronic health care needs related to their disability often take precedence and routine gynaecologic care and pelvic exams may be neglected.

Many of the challenges in providing gynaecologic care to a woman with a physical disability are related to the physical space of the health care practice. Exam rooms are often small and maneuvering with a wheelchair, scooter, or other assistive devices, such as a walker, can be extremely difficult. The exam room may need to be rearranged or furniture, such as extra chairs, may need to be temporarily removed to accommodate larger equipment such as a wheelchair.

An exam table with a hydraulic lift is ideal for women who have mobility impairment. Most practices are only equipped with standard, nonadjustable exam tables that are too high for women to safely transfer from a wheelchair. If an adjustable exam table is not available, health care personnel must be aware of how to assist women with physical disabilities onto standard exam tables. Once on the examination table, a woman with mobility impairment may need handrails and adjustable footrests in order to stay safely on the table. Padded or strapped stirrups can increase comfort, especially for women with leg spasticity, weakness, contractures, and/or tremors. Women with impaired mobility should be booked for longer appointments and at a time when extra staff are available to provide assistance and ensure safety

Prior to the exam, the woman should empty her bladder either on her own or by intermittent bladder catheterization. Many women with physical disabilities cannot comfortably assume the lithotomy position that is traditionally used for pelvic exams. This position will be difficult for many women with paralysis, muscle weakness, spasticity, low muscle tone, and conditions that cause chronic pain and inflammation. Alternative positions should be considered based upon the individual woman and her specific disability. Side-lying, knee to chest, diamond shape (knees abducted and feet together, no stirrups), legs straight and extended into a V shape, and M shape (feet flat on exam table, no stirrups) are all possibilities from which women and providers can choose (see Figure 10.1).

Communication

Although many women with physical disabilities come to health care visits with a partner, family member, or other caregiver, it should not

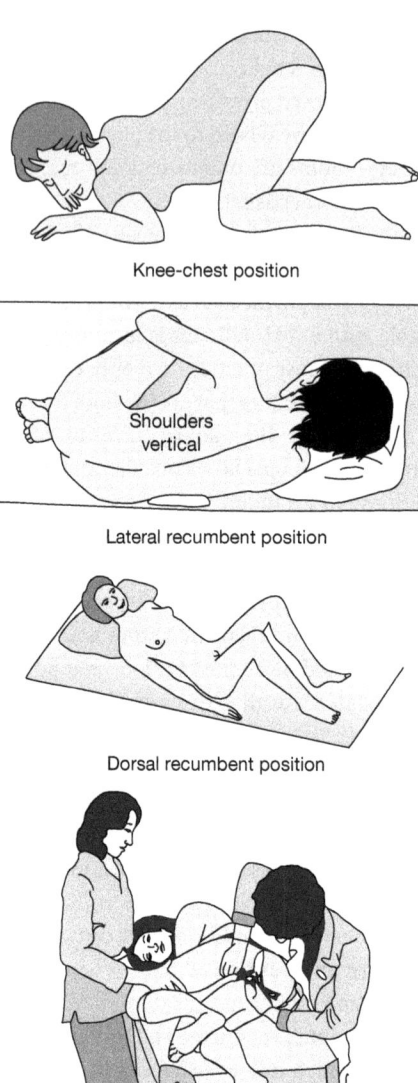

Figure 10.1 Illustrations of alternate positioning.

be assumed that the disabled woman is unable to speak for herself. Communication with women who are physically challenged should always be specifically directed to them. Other support persons may be present during conversations, but should not be used as interpreters or health care decision makers unless this is explicitly stated by the woman.

ESSENTIAL FACTS

Documentation
- Always document precautions used to ensure safety. Examples:
  - Two-person assist for transfer from wheelchair (or chair) to exam table; table set and locked to lowest position.
  - Medical assistant present during exam and to assist with positioning on and off exam table.
- Documentation should include exam findings and the woman's ability to tolerate the exam. Examples:
  - Patient unable to place legs in stirrups. Exam performed with legs flat on exam table extended into a V shape.
  - Pelvic exam limited by pain and muscle spasticity.
  - Patient tolerated exam well without hypotension or syncope.

Communication should flow normally as it would with women who are not disabled. Let the woman know the office staff and the clinician are available for assistance, but do not assume that she is unable to care for herself. Ask direct, matter-of-fact questions if there is something of which you are unsure. If assistive equipment needs to be moved in the exam room because of space constraints, the clinician should seek permission prior to relocating any devices. Moving equipment may place it out of reach and result in a risk for fall or injury if the woman is unaware of the change.

Never assume that a woman who is physically challenged is not sexually active solely because of her disability. These women need *to be asked* the same sexual history screening questions as women who are not disabled (see Chapter 1 for how to conduct a sexual history). If sexually active, type of sexual activity; number of partners; whether partners are men, women, or both; risk for pregnancy and sexually transmitted infections (STIs) and any reproductive health concerns need to be assessed. Asking direct questions such as, "Do you have any questions or concerns about your sexual health that I can help you with today?" will allow for open dialogue that will lay the foundation for a thorough gynaecologic exam.

Follow-Up

During the course of the visit, it may become apparent that follow-up is recommended based on exam findings. The clinician's assessment may reveal complications related to the disability such as pain, muscle atrophy, skin breakdown, or excoriation from prosthetic devices. If any of the clinician's findings are chronic problems, the woman should be advised to continue regular health care and monitor for worsening symptoms. New-onset symptoms, whether related to the disability or of gynaecologic origin, should be assessed more immediately. A plan for follow-up should be agreed on with the woman, and referrals implemented as necessary. Routine screening, such as mammograms and blood work, should be scheduled with facilities that are able to easily accommodate women with physical challenges.

ESSENTIAL FACTS

- Preparation of the woman, staff, space, and equipment are all necessary to ensure a safe and adequate exam for women with physical disabilities.
- Be familiar with alternate positions for performing a pelvic exam.

For further information related to specific pelvic exam challenges and potential resolutions, please see Appendix A.

11

Special Considerations When Examining the Postmenopausal and Older Woman

Heidi Collins Fantasia

Performing a gynaecologic exam on postmenopausal and elderly women requires special skills and knowledge of the physical, psychological, and social changes pertinent to this population. These include awareness of atrophic and age-related genital and pelvic exam findings. In addition, practitioners must be sensitive to other changes associated with aging, including decreased mobility, existing chronic health conditions, cognitive impairment, and impairment in eyesight and hearing.

In this chapter, you will learn how to:

- Identify normal aging changes of the vulva and vagina
- Identify atrophic changes associated with menopause
- Recognize challenges to examining postmenopausal women and identify approaches to managing the pelvic exam

EXAMINING THE POSTMENOPAUSAL AND OLDER WOMAN

Estrogen deficiency is present in all postmenopausal women. The genital skin and vaginal lining are estrogen dependent. Therefore, menopause and aging produce changes in the urogenital system that includes a shift in vaginal flora/environment, a thinning of the vaginal tissue, loss of elasticity, and urinary complaints. These changes increase the likelihood that the pelvic exam will be uncomfortable. As a result, clinicians must approach the pelvic exam with care and sensitivity.

Medical problems associated with menopause and aging may include (Carcio & Secor, 2010):

- Cardiovascular conditions such as heart attack or stroke
- Diabetes mellitus: metabolic syndrome
- Osteoporosis or osteopenia
- Asthma
- Cancers of the reproductive tract
- Sexually transmitted infections (STIs)
- Distressing vasomotor symptoms (VMS)
- Adverse effects of traditional and alternative therapies
- Gallbladder disease

AGE-RELATED AND ATROPHIC CHANGES

Certain changes associated with the loss of estrogen are identifiable when performing a gynaecologic exam on an older or elderly woman. Age-related changes of the external genitalia include thinning and graying of pubic hair, and thinning and dryness of external genital skin.

Internally, atrophic vaginitis may be evident. Inflammation from loss of estrogen can manifest as vaginal dryness, tissue pallor or erythema, loss of overall vaginal tone, decreased vaginal rugae, and loss of tissue elasticity. Cystocele and rectocele may be present. Discharge associated with atrophic vaginitis may be scant or copious, thin or thick, white or yellow, and may be associated with odor. The cervix of postmenopausal women may also lose some definition and appear flat and short. Friability and bleeding with Papanicolaou (Pap) smears are common, and often the cervical os is stenotic, which can make endocervical sampling for Pap testing challenging.

Age-related changes are also evident during the bimanual pelvic exam. Overall, pelvic reproductive organs atrophy. The uterus may be small and less mobile. If the uterus is enlarged, this may suggest pregnancy (if perimenopausal) or pathology such as uterine hyperplasia, fibroids, or carcinoma. The ovaries of a postmenopausal or elderly woman are generally not palpable, but, if palpable, the clinician should investigate further to rule out pathology by ultrasound or other imaging, cancer antigen 125 (CA125) test, and possible consultation/referral to a gynaecologist. A comparative summary of findings associated with atrophic vaginitis and other vaginal infections is presented in Table 11.1.

THE PELVIC EXAM OF THE POSTMENOPAUSAL WOMAN

The atrophic changes produced by the loss of estrogen can make the pelvic exam uncomfortable for the woman and challenging for the clinician. Age-related changes, such as decreased range of motion, arthritis, and mobility impairments, can limit positioning on the exam table. Any cognitive impairments and/or sensory impairments of sight and hearing can decrease the ability to follow directions and cooperate with the exam process. Assistance from additional staff may be needed to help with positioning on the exam table, patient safety, leg support, and obtaining specimens. If mobility and flexibility are extremely limited, the provider can perform a partial exam with the woman in the left lateral position with the right knee flexed (Sim's position).

The need for gentleness cannot be overemphasized, especially during the speculum exam. Quick insertion of the speculum and vigorous movements can be painful and damaging to thin, friable tissues. The blades of the speculum should be opened slowly and carefully to avoid vaginal tissue damage, irritation, and bleeding. Using a smaller Pederson speculum with narrower blades is often more comfortable for older women. If vaginal dryness is making speculum insertion very painful or impossible, placing a small amount of lubricant on the tip of the blades will make insertion and movement of the speculum easier. If atrophy is so significant that the pelvic exam is impossible, local application of topical estrogen (either externally or vaginally)

Table 11.1

Comparative Assessment Findings: Atrophic Vaginitis Versus Bacterial Vaginosis (*Gardnerella*)

Atrophic vaginitis	**Bacterial vaginosis**
Inspection Tissue is friable, erythema Scant, colorless discharge Sparse, brittle pubic hair Shrinking of the labia minora Possible inflammation of the vulva Vulva may be erythematous and edematous Excoriation (from vulvar pruritus)	*Inspection* Little or no inflammation of vaginal epithelium Associated with a pink, healthy cervix [Note: "Strawberry cervix" is seen with cervicitis due to *Trichomonas vaginalis*; red, edematous, friable cervix is associated with *Chlamydia trachomatis*]
Speculum exam Thin, pale, erythematous, friable vaginal epithelium Decreased or absent vaginal rugae Scant, thin, variable, nonmalodorous discharge Vaginal pH greater than 4.6 Amine test negative Microscopy: negative for clue cells, positive for WBCs, and immature epithelial cells; also referred to as an *abnormal maturation index diagnostic of atrophic vaginitis*	*Speculum exam* Homogeneous, malodorous, white, adherent vaginal discharge Vaginal pH greater than 4.6 (take smear for testing from the lateral walls of the vagina, not from the cervix) Fishy, amine-like odor from vaginal fluid before and/or after mixing it with 10% potassium hydroxide (positive whiff test) [Note: Semen releases the vaginal amines; therefore, there is an increased odor after intercourse] Presence of "clue cells" (squamous vaginal epithelial cells covered with bacteria, causing a stippled or granular appearance, and ragged, "moth-eaten" borders)

WBCs, white blood cells.

Source: Adapted with permission from Cash and Glass (2010).

can be tried for 2 to 4 weeks (or longer, if necessary) and the exam attempted again after treatment.

After menopause, the cervix may lose its landmarks and become difficult to visualize as it shortens and becomes flush with the vaginal walls. In addition, the cervical os may become smaller and stenosed, making it difficult to obtain an adequate sample for Pap smear testing. If Pap smear testing is warranted based on age and history, the clinician should insert the cytobrush approximately 1 cm into the os or as far as possible without force or trauma to the cervical canal. If a traditional Pap smear cannot be obtained, a blind Pap with human papillomavirus (HPV) DNA testing can be considered, especially for women who are at low risk for cervical cancer. Lack of estrogen makes the cervix friable and associated bleeding with cervical and endocervical sampling is not uncommon. See Chapter 1 for current Pap smear screening guidelines and recommendations for discontinuation of testing.

Other aspects of the pelvic exam may also be challenging. The bimanual exam may be limited by not only atrophic changes but also central obesity, which is common in postmenopausal women. Because of atrophy and decreased elasticity, the bimanual exam may be uncomfortable. The clinician may only be able to introduce one finger into the vagina. Palpate the uterus for shape and size. The uterus usually decreases in size after menopause as a result of atrophy. Therefore, enlargement or an irregular shape require additional evaluation. A summary of exam findings for women using and not using local estrogen is presented in Table 11.2.

Table 11.2

Assessment Findings of the Postmenopausal Woman: Using and Not Using Local Estrogen

Findings of area assessed

Findings if *not* using local estrogen	Findings if using local estrogen
External genitalia	*External genitalia*
Thinning and/or graying of pubic hair	Tissues pink, moist
Tissue pallor	Landmarks stable
Loss of architectural features (landmarks)	Elastic, durable tissues
	Nontender
Erythema	No caruncle
Easily traumatized (lesions or fissures)	Introitus normal size, with moderate tone
Tenderness	
Urethral caruncle (small friable polyp)	Stable or improving cystocele, rectocele
Introital shrinkage or laxity	
Cystocele	
Rectocele	

(continued)

Table 11.2

Assessment Findings of the Postmenopausal Woman: Using and Not Using Local Estrogen (*continued*)

Findings of area assessed

Findings if *not* using local estrogen	Findings if using local estrogen
Vagina	*Vagina*
Introital laxity	Improving introital tone
Loss of rugae (flattening)	Rugations present
Loss of tone with Kegel and Valsalva maneuvers	Improved tone with Kegel and Valsalva maneuvers
Shortening of vagina	Normal vaginal size and elasticity
Cervix	*Cervix*
Erythema	Pink
Lesions	No lesions
Friability	Nonfriable
Bleeding	Nontender
Tenderness	Less flattening with extended use
Flattening	Normal cervical os size (with continued use)
Shortening	
Stenosis of cervical os (small)	
Uterus	*Uterus*
Size and shape may be asymmetrical (associated with fibroids that shrink in menopause)	Local estrogen does not influence uterus size or shape
Diffuse enlargement (associated with pathology such as hyperplasia)	Systemic estrogen for hot flashes may cause fibroids to grow
Tenderness	
Sometimes fibroids	
Pelvic floor	*Pelvic floor*
Cystocele	Stable or improving cystocele, rectocele
Rectocele	
Diminished introital tone with Kegel and Valsalva maneuvers	Improved introital tone with Kegel and Valsalva maneuvers
Ovaries	*Ovaries*
Not palpable	Not palpable

Source: Adapted with permission from Carcio and Secor (2010).

HEALTH ISSUES OF OLDER WOMEN

In addition to the specific gynaecologic changes associated with menopause and aging, older women can experience a wide variety of health issues related to the aging process. These chronic illnesses can have a significant impact on quality of life and are a major contributor to the morbidity and mortality of older women.

- Cardiovascular disease is a broad heading that includes specific illnesses such as hypertension, cerebral vascular accidents (CVAs), congestive heart failure (CHF), and coronary artery disease (CAD). Cardiovascular disease remains the leading cause of death among women. Symptoms of acute myocardial infarction (MI) in women often present as more subtle symptoms of left arm and jaw discomfort rather than the substernal chest pain experienced by men.
- Cancer is still primarily a disease associated with aging; the vast majority of all cancers are diagnosed at age 55 or older. Breast, lung, and colorectal cancers are the most common cancers among women, with lung cancer having the highest mortality rate. Strategies for prevention and early diagnosis focus on healthy lifestyle changes and routine screening, such as mammograms and colonoscopy.
- Diabetes in older women is primarily adult onset, or type 2 diabetes mellitus. This form of diabetes is characterized by a decreased sensitivity to insulin. Type 2 diabetes is often preventable with weight reduction and increased physical activity, and is treated with lifestyle and dietary changes and medication. As the presence of diabetes increases the risk for cardiovascular disease, women should be strongly encouraged to closely manage their diabetes.
- Osteoporosis, the loss of bone density, is estimated to affect up to 20% of women older than 50 years of age and is a major contributor to hip fractures in older women. The decrease in estrogen that occurs with menopause is the leading cause of osteoporosis in women. Fractures, especially of the hip and vertebra, are often the first symptom of the disease and cause significant morbidity and mortality among older women.

LABORATORY EVALUATION OF POSTMENOPAUSAL AND OLDER WOMEN

There is no specific set of "menopause labs" that is appropriate for every woman. The decision to assess certain laboratory functions will be made based on each individual woman's history and presenting symptoms. Some laboratory tests to consider are specific to the menopause transition, whereas others relate to diseases that are more common with aging and loss of estrogen and progesterone.

- Serum follicle-stimulating hormone (FSH) is the test most commonly associated with diagnosing menopause, but it is not without controversy. A normal FSH range for menstruating women is typically between 4 and 21 mIU/mL, although this may differ slightly among laboratories. When FSH levels rise above 30, women are considered to be in menopause, but levels can fluctuate and a diagnosis of menopause cannot be made solely on one laboratory value. A clinical history of 12 consecutive months of amenorrhea is diagnostic of menopause and FSH levels are not needed to confirm clinical data.
- Estradiol is primarily made by the ovaries and decreases as ovarian function declines and eventually stops with menopause. There is a wide range for estradiol levels depending on menstrual-cycle phase, but levels less than 30 pg/mL are associated with menopause.
- Thyroid-stimulating hormone (TSH) is commonly measured to evaluate thyroid functioning. The incidence of hypothyroidism increases with age and it is estimated that up to 10% of women experience hypothyroidism by age 65. TSH is often measured to rule out a thyroid disorder as the cause of irregular menses and amenorrhea that occur with menopause.
- Luteinizing hormone (LH) is released by the pituitary gland and, in menstruating women, increases during the middle of the menstrual cycle to trigger ovulation. Normal levels range from 5 to 25 IU/L. During menopause, LH levels rise as ovarian function declines and the ovaries are less responsive to LH surges.
- Other laboratory tests to consider as women age are fasting lipid profile (FLP) and blood glucose. These tests are important in

assessing risk factors for cardiovascular disease. Bone mineral density (BMD) testing and mammogram screenings should be performed according to established guidelines and individual risk factors.

ESSENTIAL FACTS

Documentation

- Documentation should focus on physical findings related to menopause. Examples:
  - Vagina atrophic, pale, dry; decreased rugation.
  - Uterus small, smooth, mobile, nontender; ovaries nonpalpable.

Communication

Women should be reassured that the transition to menopause is a normal and expected life transition and not a pathologic state. Not all women will experience physical and emotional symptoms related to menopause. Anticipatory guidance will help dispel myths and misconceptions about menopause and aging. If women are concerned about menopause symptoms, they should be informed about pharmacologic and alternative therapies that are available to decrease discomfort, primarily from vasomotor instability.

Follow-Up

There is no specific follow-up required if the exam is normal and the woman has no immediate concerns. Menstrual calendars can be a useful tool to help women track their menstrual cycles as changes occur during the transition to menopause. A pelvic ultrasound can be considered to assess pelvic anatomy if the exam is suggestive of uterine fibroids or an ovarian mass. If perimenopausal menstrual bleeding is excessive, there is a concern about endometrial hyperplasia, or the woman complains of abnormal vaginal bleeding especially after menopause (occurring after 12 months since last menstrual period [LMP]), the woman should have an endometrial biopsy or be referred for one. A transvaginal ultrasound may also be considered.

ESSENTIAL FACTS

- Having the woman apply daily estrogen to the external genital area for 4 to 6 weeks prior to the exam may decrease discomfort by increasing elasticity and decreasing friability of the vaginal tissues.
- Using a long, narrow Pederson or pediatric speculum will decrease discomfort.
- For women who are extremely uncomfortable, applying a small amount of lidocaine gel to the vaginal introitus a few minutes prior to the exam may be beneficial.
- Use slow, gentle movements to decrease the chance of trauma with the exam.

For further information related to specific pelvic exam challenges and potential resolutions, please see Appendix A.

References

Carcio, H. A., & Secor, M. C. (2010). *Advanced health assessment of women: Clinical skills and procedures* (2nd ed.). New York, NY: Springer Publishing.

Cash, J. C., & Glass, C. A. (2010). *Family practice guidelines* (2nd ed.). New York, NY: Springer Publishing.

12

Care of the Woman Who Has Experienced Female Genital Mutilation

Heidi Collins Fantasia

Female genital mutilation (FGM), also called *female circumcision* or *female cutting*, is defined by the World Health Organization (WHO) as any procedure that involves partial or complete removal of the external female genitalia or injury to the female genitals for non-medical reasons. It is estimated that 100 to 140 million women worldwide have experienced some type of FGM and millions more are at risk. Although this practice occurs globally, it is most common in African, Middle Eastern, and some Asian countries. FGM is illegal in the United States, but practitioners may encounter women who have immigrated to the United States after having the procedure in their native country as a child.

In this chapter, you will learn how to:

- Identify different classifications of FGM
- Recognize the long-term sequelae of FGM
- Employ strategies for performing a pelvic exam after FGM

CLASSIFICATION OF FGM

The WHO has classified FGM into four categories that are based on the extent of damage to the genitalia.

- Type I involves removal of the clitoris and/or prepuce.
- Type II involves removal of the clitoris plus partial or total removal of the labia minora and possibly the labia majora.
- Type III mutilation narrows the vaginal opening by sealing over the orifice with tissue from the labia minora or majora and may also include removal of the clitoris. This level of mutilation always involves suturing that reduces the size of the vaginal introitus and often the urethral opening as well.
- Type IV includes any other harmful procedures to the female genitals that are not medically necessary. Examples include piercing, burning, scarring, or other nontherapeutic and unnecessary incisions.

ESSENTIAL FACTS

The level of anatomical alteration will differ depending on the type of FGM.

LONG-TERM SEQUELAE OF FGM

The majority of FGM occurs in young girls prior to or at the onset of puberty. Therefore, most practitioners in the United States will not experience acute cases. Rather, they will encounter women in the clinical setting long after the procedure has been performed and healing has occurred. These encounters may occur as part of a routine visit, or women may seek care because of an ongoing complication from the procedure.

- With type I and II FGM procedures, the level of scarring will vary depending on the individual woman and the conditions and instruments used in the initial procedure (Figure 12.1).

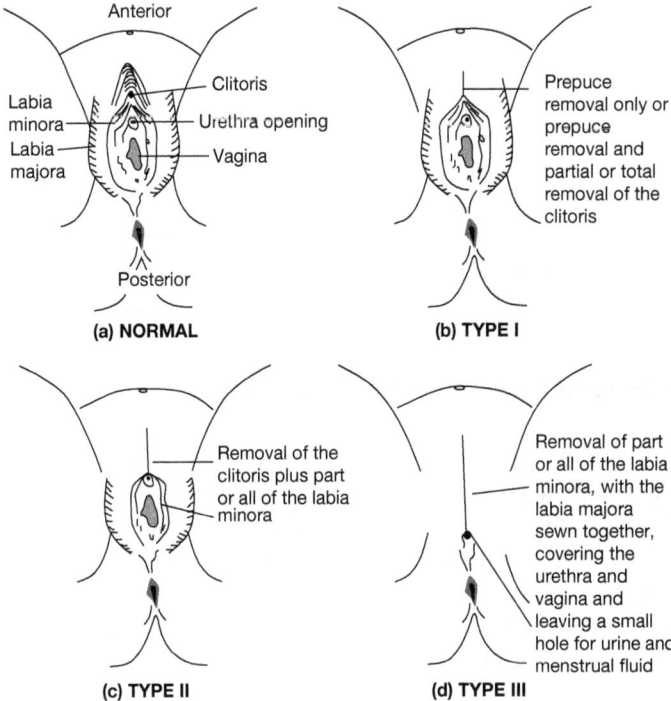

Figure 12.1 Female genital mutilation classifications.

- Possible physical symptoms include large keloid scars and epidermal inclusion cysts. Abscess formation along the scar line will present as a painful enlarging mass in the genital area.
- Some possible presenting symptoms include complaints of friable or pruritic vulvar skin that is prone to excoriation and infection and dyspareunia.
■ With type III FGM, a common gynaecologic complaint is dysmenorrhea and symptoms related to the narrowed vaginal opening. These can be grouped into the following categories:
  - Narrowing of the vaginal opening.
    ◦ Hematocolpos. This buildup of menstrual blood in the vagina results from mechanical obstruction of menstruation. Women with this condition may present with complaints of intermittent abdominal pain, constipation,

urinary retention, and complaints of vulvar pressure and bulging in the vaginal area.
- Sexual problems. Women may relate unsuccessful attempts at vaginal intercourse, infertility, sexual dysfunction, and severe dyspareunia.
- History of chronic vaginitis and pruritus.
- Narrowing of the urethral opening.
  - Women with this condition might relate a variety of urinary complaints, including prolonged voiding time, history of urinary tract infections, weak urinary flow, and dysuria.

PERFORMING A PELVIC EXAM AFTER FGM

Performing a pelvic exam on a woman who has undergone FGM requires extra time and sensitivity. A thorough reproductive history should include a discussion of any previous or current sexual activity or attempts at sexual activity. Depending on the level of alteration and scarring, successful vaginal penetration may not be possible or may be possible only in the presence of severe dyspareunia. Characteristics of menstrual and urinary flow will help determine whether vaginal and urinary openings have been significantly narrowed. The clinician should also inquire about any history of vaginal pain, itching, or sexually transmitted infections (STIs).

An external exam will reveal altered anatomy and scarring, and clinical anatomical landmarks may be difficult to identify or be completely absent. Determining how much the woman understands about the level of genital modification will help the clinician guide the flow of the pelvic exam. The type of FGM will guide how to proceed with an internal exam.

ESSENTIAL FACTS

Depending on the age of the woman when FGM was performed, she may or may not have a complete understanding of the extent of her injuries. If she was raised in an environment where all women have experienced FGM, she may have never seen unaltered female anatomy.

If the vaginal introitus is extremely narrow, pelvic exams may be difficult or impossible. A thin adult speculum or a pediatric speculum may be necessary when obtaining a Papanicolaou (Pap) smear. If the woman cannot tolerate even the smallest speculum, the Pap smear and other cervical and vaginal samples (for STIs and vaginitis) can be collected with a blind sweep. STIs and pregnancy may also be ruled out by urine testing. Assessing internal pelvic organs with a bimanual exam may also be very limited or impossible because of pain; in this situation, a pelvic ultrasound may be helpful.

Strategies to help reduce discomfort during the exam include:

- Encouraging the woman to employ deep-breathing techniques
- Use of slow, gentle movements by the examiner
- Application of topical lubricants and lidocaine to the area prior to the exam

Although such strategies can be effective in reducing discomfort during a pelvic exam, these approaches may be of limited effectiveness in the presence of significantly altered anatomy.

ESSENTIAL FACTS

Documentation

- In addition to documenting any adverse symptoms, it is important to describe exam findings in great detail. Although it may not be possible to determine the exact level of FGM, a clear description of anatomical findings is necessary to establish a plan of care. Examples:
  - Clitoris absent, well-healed scar.
  - Labia minora absent, urethral and vaginal openings patent without narrowing or scar tissue.
- The woman's response to the pelvic exam should be noted. Examples:
  - Able to insert narrow speculum but unable to open blades because of patient discomfort.
  - Bimanual exam limited by vaginal stricture and patient discomfort.

Communication

Culturally sensitive and respectful communication is essential when caring for women who have experienced FGM. This practice, although widely considered a human rights violation, is deeply rooted in culture and tradition in some areas of the world. Regarded as a rite of passage for young girls, FGM is thought to be performed to preserve purity and virginity prior to marriage, promote cleanliness, decrease promiscuity, or uphold cultural and religious traditions of a community. Families of young girls are often under great pressure to conform to local, cultural norms and risk being ostracized and/or having their daughters labeled as ineligible for marriage if FGM is not performed according to local traditions.

When discussing issues relating to sexual and reproductive health, clinicians must first determine the individual woman's feelings toward the procedure. The term *mutilation* is commonly used in Western culture to describe the level of alteration to the genitals, but some women may find this term offensive, especially if they view FGM as an important aspect of womanhood within their culture. Some women may prefer the term *cutting* when speaking of having the procedure done. Not all women will view FGM as abnormal and therefore may not be interested in genital reconstruction.

Follow-Up

Depending of the level of FGM, results of the exam, and reason for the visit, some women may require a referral for surgical evaluation. Defibulation is the process of reconstructive surgery to open the scar that narrows the vaginal and urinary openings. Common reasons for requesting defibulation include a desire for pregnancy and vaginal delivery, relief from dyspareunia, and correction of urinary and menstrual difficulties. Referral for gynaecologic evaluation under anesthesia may be necessary if the woman presents with symptoms that cannot be adequately diagnosed in a routine office visit. It is imperative to take into consideration the woman's preferences and exam findings when evaluating the need for referral.

> **ESSENTIAL FACTS**
>
> It is important to recognize that some women may not want corrective surgery, even in the presence of multiple adverse symptoms.

For further information related to specific pelvic exam challenges and potential resolutions, please see Appendix A.

13

Gynaecological Examination of the Transgender Patient

Teri Bunker

Transgender and gender-nonconforming patients are at risk for human papillomavirus (HPV) and other sexually transmitted infections, but face unique barriers to receiving care. Providers can take steps to ensure that these patients receive safe, respectful, and appropriate care.

In this chapter, you will learn:

- Appropriate language to use with transgender and gender-nonconforming patients
- Appropriate gynaecological exam strategies for transgender patients
- To understand barriers to care for transgender and gender-nonconforming patients

Table 13.1

Communications Guidelines for Transgender Patients

Language to avoid	Language to use
Queer	Gay, lesbian, bisexual, or transgender
Homosexual	Gay, lesbian
Hermaphrodite	Intersex
Transvestite	Cross-dresser
Transgendered	Transgender
Transsexual	Transgender
She-male, tranny	Transgender, gender nonconforming
MTF	Transwoman
FTM	Transman
Sex reassignment surgery	Gender-affirming surgery

FTM, female to male; MTF, male to female.

HISTORY-TAKING AND COMMUNICATION CONSIDERATIONS

It is important to establish a good rapport with the patient in a gender-confirming manner, as in the following (see also Tables 13.1 through 13.3):

- Ask for and address patients by their preferred name and pronoun.
- Use the preferred name and pronoun when speaking with or about patients and when documenting their care in the medical record.
- Be aware of your own body language—do not show surprise, shock, dismay, or concern when you discover that your patient is transgender. The patient has likely had many experiences of being asked inappropriate or insensitive questions.
- Ask questions that are pertinent to the reason for the visit and appropriate medical history.

Gender Terms

Personal gender identity can vary along a spectrum, some may reject the traditional binary gender construct entirely and others may identify strongly as male or female, as follows:

- Individuals who identify with their assigned sex at birth are cisgender, whereas those who identify as the opposite gender assigned at birth are transgender.
- Those born with an intersex chromosomal condition may be assigned a gender at birth that does not resonate with them as they mature and form their own gender identity.
- Others do not identify with any specific gender and may choose to identify as nonbinary or genderqueer.
- *It is important to ask patients their gender identity and to respect their own gender identity at all times.*

Sex, Sexual Orientation, Gender Identity, and Gender Expression

Sex is assigned at birth based on the appearance of the external genitalia. When an intersex condition is noted at birth, sex is often chosen or assigned at birth, which may or may not resonate as true for the individual later in life.

Sexual orientation describes the sexual and romantic attractions of an individual from a gender-identity perspective. A person may be sexually attracted to someone who is the same gender, the opposite gender, or all genders. For example, a person may be assigned as male at birth, be only sexually attracted to females (i.e., be considered heterosexual), and then transition to female. After transition the person may continue to be sexually attracted exclusively to females (i.e., now considered lesbian). Sexual orientation is not dependent upon, nor is it a predictor of one's gender identity.

Gender identity is one's self-identified conception of self. A person may identity as male or female, a blend of male *and* female, or as genderless.

Gender expression is the gender presentation/gender role (hairstyle, clothing choice, behaviors) chosen by a person based on societal expectations of what is deemed to be appropriately masculine or feminine. Individuals who do not express their gender within the expected societal norms are considered gender nonconforming.

TECHNIQUES OF PHYSICAL EXAMINATION

The physical examination of the patient should be relevant to the existing anatomy of the patient, regardless of gender presentation.

Conduct a careful history to elicit the information needed to guide your physical examination. If an individual has a particular body part or organ that otherwise meets the criteria for screening based on risk factors or symptoms, screening should commence regardless of hormone use. (See Table 13.3 for further guidance on facilitating the patient experience.)

Transwoman

A vaginal exam on a transgender woman is best done using an anoscope. The neovagina created in a transwoman is different than a natal vagina in that it contains a blind cuff, and lacks a cervix and surrounding fornices. The likelihood of cancer is low in the neovagina unless the tip of the penis was used to create a cervix. There is no need for routine Papanicolaou (Pap) smears or vaginal wall sampling of the neovagina unless the patient has pain or bleeding.

Transman

Do not assume anything about sexual orientation or the type of sexual activities in which the patient engages. Ask the patient specific questions such as: "What are the genders of your sexual partners?" Ask specific questions as needed to clarify the type of sexual activity the patient engages in.

The patient may prefer you use nonmedical terms for body parts. Ask the patient ahead of time what the preferred words for body parts are. Some might prefer to refer to their vagina as their "front" or "front hole."

- If the patient has a uterus and has sex with cismen ask what contraceptives are used. (Testosterone is not a sufficient contraceptive method.)
- Ask whether they have penetrative sex; this may help you to gauge the comfort level for a pelvic exam.
- Explain exactly what a Pap test is if they have never had one before. Show them the speculum and explain the procedure to them and why it is necessary.

The pelvic exam for a transman may be emotionally traumatic and may trigger dysphoria because of its association with a woman's wellness exam. Talk to the patient about HPV risk and that the exam is a screening test for cancer for men and women. When working with a new patient, it might be necessary to establish a trusting relationship over the course of several visits before doing a pelvic exam.

- Ask the patient whether they would like you to explain the procedure to them ahead of time.
- Ask about past experiences and ask whether there is anything you can do to make the procedure more comfortable for them or whether they would like to have a friend or partner present for the exam.
- Avoid bringing students into these exams as patients may be made even more uncomfortable and be made to feel like they are curiosities.

Additional considerations:

- Transmen are much less likely to be up to date on cervical cancer screening and have a higher rate of inadequate specimen collection.
- It is important to note explicitly on the laboratory report that the sample was taken from the cervix, especially if the gender marker on the patient chart or insurance information indicates the person is male, lest the laboratory discard the specimen erroneously believing there was a mistake.
- Note the use of testosterone or amenorrhea on the specimen form.
- Be prepared to advocate with the insurance company if the insurance company denies the claim.
- The insurance claim status may trigger gender dysphoria for the patient during subsequent visits.

Consider offering an external exam and/or bimanual exam as an initial step and as a way to establish trust for future exams. If the patient is unable to tolerate a pelvic exam using a speculum, consider self-collection for HPV testing. Research is lacking regarding the adequacy and reliability of self-collected HPV and Pap tests but it may be better than foregoing the test all together. Hormone treatment should never be delayed or withheld contingent upon obtaining a Pap smear.

Testosterone causes vaginal atrophy and dryness. The use of vaginal estrogens for 1 to 2 weeks prior to the exam may decrease vaginal

Table 13.2

Nongendered Language and Terms

Instead of	Use instead
Vulva	Front part, pelvic area, outer parts
Labia	Outer folds
Vagina	Front opening, front hole, inner canal
Uterus/ovaries	Internal parts
Breasts	Chest
Pap smear	Cancer or HPV screen
Bra/panties	Underwear
Pads/Tampons	Absorbent products
Period/menses	Bleeding
Stirrups	Footrests
Statements such as "I'm going to stick it in you" or "You're going to feel a little poke"	"You're going to feel me touching you" or "You're going to feel the speculum now"

HPV, human papillomavirus; Pap, Papanicolaou.

atrophy related to testosterone use, although discuss this with the patient as they may be averse to taking any estrogen even for a short time. The use of warm water and lubricant or a little lidocaine jelly for speculum insertion can make insertion much more comfortable. The genitals of a transmale who is on testosterone may look different; clitoromegaly and atrophy of the cervix and the vaginal walls are normal findings.

Anal Pap

Men who engage in receptive anal sex with other men are in a high-risk group for anal cancer; as such, transwomen may be particularly at high risk. An anal Pap should be considered for all patients who engage in receptive anal sex. The rectal mucosa is highly receptive to sexually transmitted infections, including HPV, gonorrhea, and chlamydia.

Rectal chlamydia and gonorrhea can be diagnosed by testing a rectal swab specimen with nucleic acid amplification tests (NAATs). NAATs are not FDA (Food and Drug Administration) approved for

Table 13.3

Facilitating the Patient Experience

- Transgender-friendly providers are listed on health-finder websites such as Gay and Lesbian Medical Association (GLMA), Human Rights Campaign (HRC).
- Provide waiting area periodicals such as *The Advocate* or HRC publications or brochures.
- Avoid asking unnecessary questions. Before asking the question, ask yourself whether you are asking out of your own curiosity or if the answer is important to the patient's care.
- Use gender-neutral pronouns; ask for preferred name and avoid using Mr./Ms./Miss/Mrs.
- Ask the patient about preferred pronouns and terms for body parts.
- Apologize if you make a mistake and use the wrong pronoun.
- Have gender-neutral bathrooms.
- Display nondiscriminatory policies.
- Have trans-inclusive options on patient registration forms.
- Explain the exam in nonsexualized and nongendered terms using the patient's preferred language.

During and after the exam:

- Use a small or pediatric speculum, using a water-based or topical lidocaine lubricant.
- Sample a greater portion of the cervix to ensure adequacy of cells.
- Avoid comments about genitals.
- Consider collecting cervical cells with a vaginal swab if a pelvic exam is not possible.
- Warn about possible bleeding.
- Advise that there is always a possibility that the sample is inadequate and may need retesting in 2–4 months.
- Ensure that patient has a support system if needed for postexam care.

---

rectal testing, but may be used by labs that have met the regulatory requirements. The best way to screen for anal HPV is by sampling the cells of the anus with a Pap smear.

The steps for performing an anal Pap are as follows:

- Patients are asked to not douche, use an enema, or insert anything into the anus for 24 hours prior to the exam.
- Position the patient in a comfortable position that allows access to the anus.
- Retract the buttocks to expose the anus.

- Insert a Dacron or polyester-tipped swab moistened with water 2 to 3 inches into the anus. Do not use a wooden-shafted swab as it may splinter.
- As you advance the swab, note the slight resistance as the swab passes through the internal sphincter, and gently advance the swab a little more to the dentate line and the transformation zone, where most HPV-related lesions are located.
- Rotate the swab 360 degrees while applying firm lateral pressure to the end of the swab, and continue to rotate and withdraw the swab slowly over a period of 15 to 30 seconds. The firm pressure on the swab ensures that you are sampling rectal cells and not the contents of the rectum.
- Liquid cytology is the preferred preservation method. The swab is vigorously agitated in the preservative solution and labeled appropriately.
- Perform a digital rectal examination and note any nodules, condyloma, or any rough-textured anal skin.
- Examine the perineal area for any grayish or hyperpigmented patches, which may indicate high-grade anal intraepithelial neoplasia (HGAIN), which is the precursor to anal cancer.

CONCLUSION

It is important that all providers work to eliminate barriers to access to care for transgender and gender-nonconforming people. It is important to create a welcoming environment and to understand the barriers to care and to become educated in the specific health care needs of this population.

Appendices

Appendix A
Common Pelvic Examination Problems and Interventions

Pelvic examination problem	Interventions
Extreme anxiety	Defer exam; palpate cervix before the bimanual exam; use step-by-step desensitization; suggest relaxation techniques and/or deep breathing; suggest antianxiety meds, counseling
Inability to insert speculum due to discomfort	Use Pederson or small speculum
	Use a swab to collect samples for Pap, STIs, wet mount; suggest deep breathing
	Consider urine testing for STIs
Inability to insert speculum due to dryness	Palpate introital tissues or cervix before speculum insertion
	Apply scant lubricant to tip of speculum
Inability to insert speculum due to small and/or tight introitus	Palpate cervix; use small Pederson speculum or Dacron swab for STIs, wet mount; suggest relaxation breathing
Inability to visualize cervix	Palpate cervix before speculum exam, move speculum side to side (shimmy), change angle slightly, instruct patient to bear down; try larger speculum, open wider

(continued)

Pelvic examination problem	Interventions
Vaginal walls impede visualizing cervix	Place condom or glove over speculum (cut off tip)
	Use larger blade speculum like Graves or Clinton Graves; open wide
	Use Guttman or "Snowman" lateral vaginal wall retractor
Inability to view cervix because of extreme posterior position	Use large, extra-long speculum like the "Clinton Pederson" style; open wide; palpate cervix before, push down on suprapubic area, instruct patient to bear down, lift hips, spread thighs, and rest their bent knees on knee stirrups
Speculum comes out unless clinician holds it	Seek an assistant to hold the speculum while you collect specimens, remove speculum, then prepare tests
Patient unable to tolerate speculum in situ secondary to anxiety and/or pain	Collect samples, remove speculum, then prepare tests
	Remember, samples are stable on sampling tools
History of physical or sexual abuse and extreme phobia of pelvic exams—with or without vaginismus	Comanage with a specialized counselor; use step-by-step desensitization program; may not be able to complete a pelvic exam for several visits (may take months or years)

Pap, Papanicolaou; STIs, sexually transmitted infections.

©Mimi Secor, 2017. (May be copied but not altered.)

Appendix B
Vaginal Microscopy Flow Sheet

Date			
History of present illness (HPI)			
LMP, last coitus			
Vulva, vagina, cervix			
Vaginal mucus			
Cervical mucus			
pH (4.0–7.5) <4.7 = normal			
Amine test (KOH)			
Wet mount (saline)			
Low power (quality) Properly prepared smear?			
High power (detail)			
Lactobacilli (LB) (0–3+)			
Bacteria (0–3+)			
WBCs (0–3+)			
Other			
Wet mount (KOH)			
Low power (hyphae and buds)			
High power			
Assessment			
Plan			

KOH, potassium hydroxide; LMP, last menstrual period; WBCs, white blood cells.

©Mimi Secor, 2017. (May be copied but not altered.)

Appendix C
Vaginal Microscopy: Flow Sheet Instructions

Date: _____

	Brief history of symptoms, including self-care, meds
LMP, last coitus	LMP, last coitus, dyspareunia
Vulva, vagina, cervix	Erythema, lesions, tenderness
Vaginal mucus	Amount and characteristics
Cervical mucus	Color, quality, amount
pH (4.0–7.5) (<4.7 = normal)	Use 1-inch strip of Nitrazine or ColorpHast paper; dip pH paper into vaginal mucus collected on spatula or swab
Amine test (10% KOH)	Using spatula with sample, stir 10 times into 20% KOH on glass slide (use two slides, one for KOH, one for saline); check fishy, foul odor
Wet mount (saline) (dilute w/ scattered epithelial cells [ECs])	Using wooden spatula containing sample, stir three times into saline solution on glass slide
Low power (quality), 10× magnification	General appearance and quality of sample, for example, proper concentration, too diluted, too concentrated

(continued)

High power (detail), 40× magnification	Identify organisms and morphology
LB (0–3+); appear as rods	1+ = few, 2 = dominant, 3+ = false clue cells
Bacteria = anaerobes (0–3+); appear as tiny cocci	1+ = few per HPF, 2+ = dominant background per HPF, 3+ = clue cells
WBCs (0–3+) size of nucleus of an EC	1+ = 1:1 ratio to ECs, 2+ = 5:1, 3+ = 10:1 or greater
Other, including ECs	ECs (true clue cells, false clue cells, superficial, parabasal, basal), yeast, trichomoniasis, mobiluncus, sperm, RBCs, medications, artifact
Wet mount (KOH; very concentrated)	ECs look like round, hollow balloons called *ghost cells*
Low power	Hyphael forms (cobwebs) visible, but not buds
High power	Hyphae look like elongated balloons; buds = spherical glass beads, slightly different sizes and shapes
Assessment	Specify, including rule-outs; list most likely to least likely
Plan	Diagnostic tests, including yeast cultures; meds; education; follow-up

HPF, high-power field; KOH, potassium hydroxide; LB, lactobacilli; LMP, last menstrual period; RBCs, red blood cells; WBCs, white blood cells.

©Mimi Secor, 2017. (May be copied but not altered.)

Appendix D
Vulvar Care Guidelines for Patient Education

- For vulvar itching
  - Hydrocortisone 1% ointment, over the counter
    - Apply twice a day as needed (no limit on how long you can use)
  - Clobetasol or halobetasol 0.05% ointment (if prescribed)
    - Apply daily for 2 weeks, then every other day for 2 to 4 weeks, then once or twice weekly as needed
  - Apply Vaseline, Crisco, or pure mineral oil daily or more often
  - Increase use of lubricants as you taper the clobetasol or hydrocortisone
- Vulvar care basics: "Less is more"—do not scrub
  - Wash with warm water
  - Avoid washing with soap
  - May use mineral or coconut oil as a soap substitute (pure unscented—not baby oil)
  - Avoid mechanical or chemical pubic hair removal: especially near the vagina—trimming hair is okay
- Wear all-cotton *or* synthetic underwear with cotton-crotch insert
  - Avoid thong underwear: may cause bacteria to move from "back to front"
  - Wash in hot water, double rinse
  - Use half the soap recommended

- Avoid intercourse during treatment and while you are having symptoms
  - Avoid sex if painful
  - Use condoms when possible
- Wipe from "front to back"
- Sex
  - Wash hands and partner's hands/penis before sex
  - Use water-based lubricants such as K-Y products
  - Unscented, unflavored, Silke, Intrigue, Slippery Stuff, Poise, Sliquid, or plain K-Y; coconut or vegetable oil is okay if not using latex condoms
  - Use condoms, especially with anal intercourse
    - Use a new condom for vaginal intercourse
    - Olive oil or commercial products are irritating
  - Wash sex toys
  - Try to maintain a similar pattern of sexual activity over time
- Avoid douching; the vagina is self-cleaning
- Reduce your stress
- Increase sleep
- Sleep without underwear; wear loose clothing during day, especially avoid tight jeans
- Return when recommended and if symptoms persist or recur

©Mimi Secor, 2017. (May be copied but not altered.)

Bibliography

Abdulcadir, J., Margairaz, C., Boulvain, M., & Irion, O. (2011). Care of women with female genital mutilation/cutting. *Swiss Medical Weekly, 140*, 1–8.

ACOG Committee on Practice Bulletins—Gynecology. (2009). ACOG Practice Bulletin No. 109: Cervical cytology screening. *Obstetrics & Gynecology, 114*, 1409–1420.

American College of Obstetricians and Gynecologists. (2012). Intimate partner violence. Retrieved from http://www.acog.org/~/media/Committee%20Opinions/Committee%20on%20Health%20Care%20for%20Underserved%20Women/co518.pdf?dmc=1&ts=20140921T13352692

American College of Obstetricians and Gynecologists. (2014). The initial reproductive health visit. Retrieved from http://www.acog.org/Resources-And-Publications/Committee-Opinions/Committee-on-Adolescent-Health-Care/The-Initial-Reproductive-Health-Visit

American Medical Association. (2008). Opinion 2.02—Physicians' obligations in preventing, identifying, and treating violence and abuse. Retrieved from https://www.ama-assn.org/sites/default/files/media-browser/public/aboutama/councils/Council%20Reports/council-on-ethics-and-judicial-affairs/i07-ceja-violence-abuse.pdf

Bates, C. K., Carroll, N., & Potter, J. (2010). The challenging pelvic examination. *Journal of General Internal Medicine, 26*(6), 651–657.

Braddy, C. M., & Files, J. A. (2007). Female genital mutilation: Cultural awareness and clinical considerations. *Journal of Midwifery and Women's Health, 52*, 158–163.

Carter, S., Rad, M., Schwarz, B., Van Sell, S., & Marshall, D. (2013). Creating a more positive patient experience of pelvic examination. *Journal of the American Association of Nurse Practitioners, 25*, 611–618.

Center of Excellence for Transgender Health. (n.d.). Retrieved from http://transhealth.ucsf.edu

Centers for Disease Control and Prevention. (2015). Sexually transmitted diseases guidelines, 2015. *Morbidity and Mortality Weekly Report, 64*(RR-3), 1–137.

Centers for Disease Control and Prevention. (2016). U.S. medical eligibility criteria for contraceptive use. *Morbidity and Mortality Weekly Report, 65*(RR-3), 1–104.

Chelmow, D., Waxman, A., Cain, J. M., & Lawrence, H. C., III. (2012). The evolution of cervical screening and the specialty of obstetrics and gynecology [Abstract]. *Obstetrics & Gynecology, 119*, 695–699.

Dahl, R. E. (2004). Adolescent brain development: A period of vulnerabilities and opportunities. *Annals of the New York Academy of Sciences, 1021*, 1–22.

The Fenway Institute. (2017). Retrieved from https://www.lgbthealtheducation.org

Fogel, C. I., & Woods, N. F. (2008). *Woman's health care in advanced practice nursing*. New York, NY: Springer Publishing.

Giadino, A. P., Datner, E. M., & Asher, J. B. (2003). *Sexual assault victimization: Across the lifespan*. St. Louis, MO: JW Medical.

Hamoudi, A., & Shier, M. (2010). Late complications of childhood female genital mutilation. *Journal of Obstetrics and Gynaecology Canada, 32*, 587–589.

Harmanli, O., & Jones, K. A. (2010). Using lubricant for speculum insertion. *Obstetrics & Gynecology, 116*, 415–417.

Hawkins, J. W., Roberto-Nichols, D. M., & Stanley-Haney, J. L. (2016). *Guidelines for nurse practitioners in gynaecologic settings* (11th ed.). New York, NY: Springer Publishing.

Hertweck, P., & Yoost, J. (2010). Common problems in pediatric and adolescent gynecology. *Expert Review of Obstetrics and Gynecology, 5*(3), 311–328.

Institute of Medicine. (2011). *Clinical preventive services for women: Closing the gaps*. Washington, DC: National Academies Press.

Jarvis, C. (2008). *Physical examination and health assessment* (5th ed.). St. Louis, MO: Saunders.

Kaul, P., Gong, J., & Guiton, G. (2014). Effective feedback strategies for teaching in pediatric and adolescent gynecology. *Journal of Pediatric and Adolescent Gynecology, 27*, 188–193.

Logan, T. K., Walker, R., & Hunt, G. (2009). Understanding human trafficking in the United States. *Trauma, Violence, and Abuse, 10*(3), 3–30. doi:10.1177/1524838008327262

Massad, L. S., Einstein, M. H., Huh, W. K., Katki, H. A., Kinney, W. K., Schiffman, M., . . . Lawson, H. W. (2013). 2012 updated consensus guidelines for the management of abnormal cervical cancer screening tests and cancer precursors. *Journal of Lower Genital Tract Disease, 17*(Suppl. 1), S1–S27.

McClain, N. M., & Garrity, S. E. (2011). Sex trafficking and the exploitation of adolescents. *Journal of Obstetrics, Gynaecologic, and Neonatal Nursing, 40*, 243–252. doi:10.1111/j.1552-6909.2011.01221.x

Momoh, C. (2010). Female genital mutilation. *Trends in Urology, Gynaecology & Sexual Health, 15*, 11–14.

Moyer, V. A. (2012). Screening for cervical cancer: US Preventive Services Task Force recommendation statement. *Annals of Internal Medicine, 156*(12), 880–891. doi:10.7326/0003-4819-156-12-201206190-00424

Nelson, A., & Rubin, M. (2011). Anal dysplasia. *Female Patient, 36*, 1–5.

Potter, J., Peitzmeirer, S. M., Reisner, S. L., Alizaga, N. M., Agenor, M., & Pardee, G. M. (2015). Cervical cancer screening for patients on the female-to-male spectrum: A narrative review and guide for clinicians. *Journal of General Internal Medicine, 30*, 1860–1861.

Quinn, G. P., Sanchez, J. A., Sutton, S. K., Vadaparampil, S. T., Nguyen, G. T., Green, B. L., . . . Schabath, M. B. (2015). Cancer and lesbian, gay, bisexual, transgender/transsexual, and queer/questioning (LGBTQ) populations. *CA: A Cancer Journal for Clinicians, 65*, 384–400. doi:10.3322/caac.21288

Richman, S. M., & Drickamer, M. A. (2007). Gynaecologic care of elderly women. *Journal of the American Medical Directors Association, 8*(4), 219–223.

Saslow, D., Solomon, D., Lawson, H. W., Killackey, M., Kulasingam, S. L., Cain, P., . . . ACS-ASCCP-ASCP Cervical Cancer Guideline Committee. (2012). American Cancer Society, American Society for Colposcopy and Cervical Pathology, and American Society for Clinical Pathology screening guidelines for the prevention and early detection of cervical cancer. *CA: A Cancer Journal for Clinicians, 62*, 147–172. doi:10.3322/caac.21139

Secor, M. (1998). The gynaecologic exam. In H. Carcio (Ed.), *Infertility for the primary care provider*. Philadelphia, PA: Lippincott-Raven.

Tanner, J. M. (1962). *Growth at adolescence*. Oxford, UK: Blackwell Scientific.

Thackeray, J. D., Hibbard, R., & Dowd, M. D. (2010). Intimate partner violence: The role of the pediatrician. *Pediatrics, 125*, 1094–1100.

Tjaden, P., & Thoennes, N. (2000). *Full report of the prevalence, incidence, and consequences of violence against women: Findings from the National Violence Against Women survey* (NCJ183781). Washington, DC: National Institute of Justice, Office of Justice Programs, U.S. Department of Justice. Retrieved from https://www.ncjrs.gov/pdffiles1/nij/183781.pdf

U.S. Cancer Statistics Working Group. (2010). *United States Cancer Statistics: 1999–2007 Incidence and mortality web-based report*. Atlanta, GA: Department of Health and Human Services, Centers for Disease Control and Prevention, and National Cancer Institute. Retrieved from http://www.cdc.gov/uscs

U.S. Department of State. (2006). *Trafficking in persons report*. Washington, DC: Author. Retrieved from https://www.state.gov/g/tip/rls/tiprpt/2006

Wee, C. C., McCartney, E. P., Davis, R. B., & Phillips, R. S. (2000). Screening for cervical and breast cancer: Is obesity an unrecognized barrier to preventive care? *Annals of Internal Medicine, 132*, 697–704.

Weitlauf, J. C., Finney, J. W., Ruzek, J., Lee, T. T., Thrailkill, A., Jones, S., & Frayne, S. M. (2008). Distress and pain during pelvic examinations: Effect of sexual violence. *Obstetrics & Gynecology, 112*, 1343–1350.

World Health Organization. (2008). *Eliminating female genital mutilation: An interagency statement*. Geneva, Switzerland: Author.

World Professional Association for Transgender Health. (2011). Standards of care for the health of transsexual, transgender, and gender nonconforming people; seventh version. Retrieved from http://www.wpath.org/site_home.cfm

RESOURCES

Cervical cancer screening guidelines
www.asccp.org
www.acog.org
www.cancer.org/health-care-professionals/american-cancer-society-prevention-early-detection-guidelines/cervical-cancer-screening-guidelines.html

Contraceptive guidelines
2016 CDC Contraceptive Medical Eligibility Criteria
www.cdc.gov/mmwr/volumes/65/rr/rr6503a1.htm

Menopause information
North American Menopause Association
www.nams.org

Sexually transmitted infections
2015 CDC STI Treatment Guidelines
www.cdc.gov/mmwr/preview/mmwrhtml/rr6403a1.htm

Abbreviations

AAP	American Academy of Pediatrics
ACOG	American College of Obstetricians and Gynecologists
AMA	American Medical Association
ASC-H	suspect high-grade lesion
ASC-US	atypical squamous cells of unclear significance
AUB	abnormal uterine bleeding
BMD	bone mineral density
BMI	body mass index
BV	bacterial vaginosis
CAD	coronary artery disease
CA125	cancer antigen 125
CBC	complete blood count
CHF	congestive heart failure
CIN	cervical intraepithelial neoplasia
CMT	cervical motion tenderness
CNS	central nervous system
CVA	cerebral vascular accidents
CVAT	costovertebral angle tenderness
DUB	dysfunctional uterine bleeding
EC	epithelial cell

EMR	electronic medical record
E-stim	electrical stimulation
FDA	Food and Drug Administration
FGM	female genital mutilation (also called *female circumcision* or *female cutting*)
FLP	fasting lipid profile
FSH	follicle-stimulating hormone
FTM	female to male
GI	gastrointestinal
GLMA	Gay and Lesbian Medical Association
HGAIN	high-grade anal intraepithelial neoplasia
HIPAA	Health Insurance Portability and Accountability Act of 1996
HPF	high-power field
HPV	human papillomavirus
HRA	high-resolution anoscopy
HRC	Human Rights Campaign
hr-HPV	high-risk human papillomavirus
HSIL	high-grade squamous intraepithelial lesion
HSV	herpes simplex virus
IgG	immunoglobulin G
IOM	Institute of Medicine
IPV	intimate partner violence
IUD	intrauterine device
KOH	potassium hydroxide
LH	luteinizing hormone
LMP	last menstrual period
LP	lichen planus
LS	lichen sclerosis
LSC	lichen simplex chronicus
LSIL	low-grade squamous intraepithelial lesion

MDL	Medical Diagnostic Laboratories
MI	myocardial infarction
MRSA	methicillin-resistant *Staphylococcus aureus*
MSM	men who have sex with men
MTF	male to female
NAAT	nucleic acid amplification testing
NSSC	normal size, shape, contour
OAB	overactive bladder
Pap	Papanicolaou
PC	pubococcygeal
PCOS	polycystic ovarian syndrome
PCR	polymerase chain reaction
PID	pelvic inflammatory disease
PUPP	pruritic urticarial papules of pregnancy
RBC	red blood cell count
ROS	review of systems
RPR	rapid plasma reagin (syphilis test)
STI	sexually transmitted infection
SV	sexual violence
TSH	thyroid-stimulating hormone
UTI	urinary tract infection
VIN	vulvar intraepithelial neoplasia
VMS	vasomotor symptoms
WBC	white blood cell
WHO	World Health Organization

Index

abdominal exam, 15–20
    assessment findings, 16–17
    gloves, 17
    order, 18, 20
    positioning, 17
    procedure, 19
    urinary tract symptoms, 18
abdominal pain, 18
adnexae, 57, 59
    assessment findings, 58
adnexal exam, 57–59
adolescents, 97–100
    brain development, 97–98
    communication, 99
    documentation, 98
    examining, 98
    follow-up, 99
age-related changes, 112–113
allodynia, 30
amine/KOH test, 48
anal cancers, 61
anal dysplasia
    anal Pap smear, 65–66
    risk factors/risk populations, 61
anal Pap smear, 134–136
    procedure, 65–66
anorectal cancer risk, 61
anoscope, 132

anteverted uterus, 54, 55
antianxiety medications, 80–81
anus, assessment findings, 27
anxiety, 80–82
    communication, 81–82
    documentation, 81
    follow-up, 82
    medications, 80–81
    relaxation techniques, 80
atrophic vaginitis, 112–113
    bacterial vaginosis versus, 114
    sticky glove test, 34

bacterial vaginosis versus atrophic vaginitis, 114
Bartholin cyst, 31
Bartholin's glands, 30–31
bimanual exam, 53–59
    adnexal exam, 57–59
    overview, 53
    uterus, 54–56
body mass index (BMI), 102
brain development, adolescents, 97–98

cancer
    cervical, 38
    neovagina and, 132
    older women, 117

155

cardiovascular disease in older women, 117
cervical cancer, screening guidelines, 38
cervix
 assessment findings, 44–45
 blue-tinged, 43
 multiparous, 46, 50
 nulliparous, 43, 46, 50
 view through speculum, 50
 visualization of, 71–73
challenging clinical situations
 visualization of cervix, 71–73
 vulvar/vaginal itching, 75–77
 vulvar/vaginal pain, 74–75
chancroid, 23. *See also* sexually transmitted infections
childbirth, pelvic muscles, 104
children, 94–97
 communication, 96
 considerations, 94
 documentation, 96
 examining, 95–96
 follow-up, 97
 obtaining history, 94
 Tanner stages, 94–95
chlamydia, 23. *See also* sexually transmitted infections
cisgender, 131
clitoris, assessment findings, 27
coitarche, 9
colonoscopy, 64
communicating role of nurse practitioner. *See* rapport building
communication
 adolescents, 99
 anxiety, 81–82
 children, 96
 female genital mutilation, 126
 human trafficking, 90
 intimate partner violence (IPV), 86
 menopause, 119
 multiparity, 105–106
 obese women, 103–104
 physically challenged women, 107, 109–110
 sexual violence, 85
 transgender patient, 130
 vulvar/vaginal itching, 76–77
 vulvar/vaginal pain, 74–75
contraceptive history, 10–11
costovertebral angle tenderness (CVAT), 18
CVAT. *See* costovertebral angle tenderness
cystocele, 28, 32, 43, 112

Dacron swab, 30
diabetes in older women, 117
differential diagnosis of vaginal infections, 49
digital rectal examination, 136
documenting gynaecologic exam, 6
dysmenorrhea, 123

ectocervix, 46
electrical stimulation (E-stim), 34
electronic medical record (EMR), 6
EMR. *See* electronic medical record
endocervix, 46
endometrial biopsy, 119
environment. *See* therapeutic environment
erythema, 75
E-stim. *See* electrical stimulation
excoriation, 75, 76. *See also* vulvar/vaginal itching
external rectal exam, 62–63

fallopian tubes, 58
female genital mutilation (FGM), 121–127
 classification of, 122
 communication, 126
 cultural sensitivity and, 126
 defined, 121
 long-term sequelae, 122–124
 pelvic exam after, 124–127

FGM. *See* female genital mutilation
fractures in older women, 117

gender expression, 131
gender identity, 130–131
general medical history, 7
genital herpes, 23, 30. *See also* sexually transmitted infections
genital injuries, 84. *See also* sexual violence
genital skin, 112
genital warts, 23. *See also* sexually transmitted infections
gonorrhea, 23. *See also* sexually transmitted infections
guaiac test, 64
gynaecologic history, 7–8

Hart's line, 29
Health Insurance Portability and Accountability Act (HIPAA), 6
HGAIN. *See* high-grade anal intraepithelial neoplasia
high-grade anal intraepithelial neoplasia (HGAIN), 136
high-risk human papillomavirus (hrHPV) infection, 61
HIPAA. *See* Health Insurance Portability and Accountability Act
hormone treatment, 133
hrHPV infection. *See* high-risk human papillomavirus infection
human trafficking, 88–91
  communication, 90
  documentation, 89
  follow-up, 90
  warning signs, 89
humor, use of. *See* rapport building
hymen, 29, 30
hytone dysfunction, 31

initial conversation. *See* rapport building
instructions, before appointment, 4
internal rectal exam, 63–64
interview. *See* medical interview
intimate partner violence (IPV), 83, 86–88. *See also* sexual violence
  communication, 86
  follow-up, 87
  screening, 86
IPV. *See* intimate partner violence
irritation, 75
itching. *See* vulvar/vaginal itching

Kegel exercises, 106

labia majora, 25, 28
labia minora, 25, 28, 29
laxity test, 32
lichen planus (LP), 28
liquid cytology, 136
lithotomy position
  physically challenged women, 107
  speculum exam, 39
lubricant, for rectovaginal exam, 63

medical history, 7
medical interview, 6–11
  contraceptive history, 10–11
  general medical history, 7
  gynaecologic history, 7–8
  Pap smear history, 10
  sexual history, 9–10
  UTI history, 10
menopause
  aging and, 112
  assessment findings, 115–116
  communication, 119
  documentation, 119
  medical problems with, 112
  transition to, 119
menstrual calendars, 119
menstrual cycles, 119
menstrual irregularities, 99

multiparity, 104–106
  challenges associated with, 104–105
  communication, 105–106
  follow-up, 106
  locating/palpating cervix, 105
multiparous women. *See* multiparity
multiple deliveries, pelvic muscles and, 104
mutilation, 126

NAATs. *See* nucleic acid amplification tests
natal vagina, 132
National Intimate Partner and Sexual Violence Survey, 83
neovagina, 132
nongendered language and terms, 135
non-Welch Allyn plastic speculum, 48
nucleic acid amplification tests (NAATs), 134, 135
nurse practitioner, communicating role of. *See* rapport building

OAB. *See* overactive bladder
obese women, 102–104
  communication, 103–104
  examination techniques, 102
  follow-up, 104
  menstrual irregularities, 104
  societal discrimination, 103
older women
  health issues of, 117
  laboratory evaluation of, 118–120
osteoporosis in older women, 117
ovaries
  bimanual examination, 57–59
  cystic enlargement, 58
overactive bladder (OAB), 34

pain
  abdominal, 18
  vulvar/vaginal, 74–75

Papanicolaou (Pap) smears, 125, 132
  anal, 65–66, 134–136
  cervical, collecting, 46–47
  friability and bleeding with, 112–113
  taking history, 10
patient education, vulvar care guidelines, 29, 145–146
pelvic exam
  adolescents, 97–100
  anxiety, 80–82
  children, 94–97
  after female genital mutilation, 124–127
  obese women, 102–104
  physically challenged women, 106–110
  postmenopausal woman, 113, 114–116
  problems and interventions, 139–140
  sexual violence, 82–88
  transman, 132–133
  vulvar/vaginal pain, 74–75
pelvic floor muscles, 34
pelvic floor rehabilitation, 34–35
pelvic inflammatory disease (PID), 24, 54. *See also* sexually transmitted infections
perimenopausal menstrual bleeding, 119
perineum, assessment findings, 27
physical violence, 82–85
physically challenged women, 106–110
  alternative positions, 107, 108
  communication, 107, 109–110
  exam room arrangement, 107
  follow-up, 110
  health care needs, 106–107
  lithotomy position, 107
PID. *See* pelvic inflammatory disease
postmenopausal women
  cervix of, 112
  health issues of, 117

ovaries of, 113
pelvic exam, 113, 114–116
pre-appointment instructions, 4
premenarchal children. *See* children
procidentia, 33
professional image, 5
pubic hair, Tanner stages, 94–95
pyelonephritis, 18

rapport building, 4–5
   communicating role of nurse practitioner, 5
   humor, use of, 5
   initial conversation, 5
rectal exam, 61–66
   anal Pap smears, 65–66
   external, 62–63
   indications, 62
   internal, 63–64
   overview, 61
   rectovaginal exam, 62, 63
rectocele, 28, 32, 43, 112
rectovaginal exam, 62, 63. *See also* rectal exam
relaxation techniques, 80
retroverted uterus, 54, 56, 62
romantic attractions, 131

screening
   IPV, 86
   sexual violence, 85, 88
sex, 131
sexual abuse/assault. *See* sexual violence
sexual attractions, 131
sexual exploitation, 88. *See also* human trafficking
sexual history, 9–10
sexual orientation, 131
sexual trafficking, 91. *See also* human trafficking
sexual violence, 82–85. *See also* intimate partner violence
   communication, 85
   documentation, 85
   follow-up, 87–88
   locations for injury, 84
   TEARS pneumonic, 84
   victims, 83
sexually transmitted infections (STIs), 23–24, 29, 124, 125
short-acting antianxiety medications, 80–81
speculum
   discarding, 51
   insertion, 41–43
   removing, 48
   selection, 39–41
   size, 40–41
speculum exam, 37–51
   collecting cervical Pap smear, 46–47
   diagnostic tests during, 48, 49
   equipment needed to perform, 37–38
   lithotomy position, 39
   overview, 37
   positioning, 39
   purpose of, 37
   suggestions reducing anxiety, 38–39
   vagina and cervix inspection, 43–46
sticky glove test, 34
STIs. *See* sexually transmitted infections
syphilis, 24. *See also* sexually transmitted infections

Tanner stages, 94–95
TEARS, 84
testosterone, vaginal atrophy and, 133, 134
therapeutic environment, 4
transgender patient, 129–136
   anal Pap, 134–136
   communications guidelines for, 130
   facilitating experience, 135
   physical examination, 131–136

transition to gynaecologic exam, 13
transman, 132–134
transvaginal ultrasound, 119
transwoman, 132
trichomoniasis, 24. *See also* sexually transmitted infections

unprotected intercourse, 8
urethral meatus, assessment findings, 27
urinary tract infections (UTIs), 10
urinary tract symptoms, 18
uterine fibroids, 55, 56
uterine prolapse, 32, 33
    first degree of, 32, 33
    fourth degree of, 33
    second degree of, 32
    third degree of, 32, 33
uterus, 54–56
    anteverted, 54, 55
    assessment findings, 58
    palpating, 54
    position, 54, 55
    prolapse. *See* uterine prolapse
    retroverted, 54, 56, 62
UTIs. *See* urinary tract infections

vagina
    assessment findings, 44–45
    bulging, 43
    visual inspection, 43
vaginal atrophy, testosterone and, 133, 134
vaginal dryness, 112
vaginal estrogens, 133, 134
vaginal exam, 132
vaginal folds, 43
vaginal infections, differential diagnosis of, 49
vaginal introital tone, 31–34
vaginal introitus, 125
    assessment findings, 27
    visual examination, 28
vaginal itching. *See* vulvar/vaginal itching
vaginal lining, 112

vaginal microscopy
    flow sheet, 141
    flow sheet instructions, 143–144
vaginal pain. *See* vulvar/vaginal pain
vaginal pH test, 48
Valsalva maneuver, 32
visualization of cervix, 71–73
vital signs, 11–13
    blood pressure, 12
    heart rate, 12
    respiratory rate, 12
    temperature, 12
    weight, 11
vulva, assessment findings, 25–26
vulvar care guidelines, for patient education, 29, 145–146
vulvar exam, 21–35
    approach, 21–22
    external examination of genitalia, 22, 25–28
    overview, 21
    palpation, 30–34
    pelvic floor rehabilitation, 34–35
    visual focus, 28–30
vulvar/vaginal itching, 75–77
    causes, 76
    communication, 76–77
    documentation, 76
    follow-up, 77
vulvar/vaginal pain, 74–75
    communication, 74–75
    documentation, 74
    follow-up, 75
vulvitis, 75
vulvodynia, 74. *See also* vulvar/vaginal pain

weight, 11. *See also* vital signs
weight bias, 102
wet mount examination, 75
WHO. *See* World Health Organization
wooden-shafted swab, 136
World Health Organization (WHO), 121, 122

FAST FACTS FOR YOUR NURSING CAREER

Choose from Over 40 Titles!

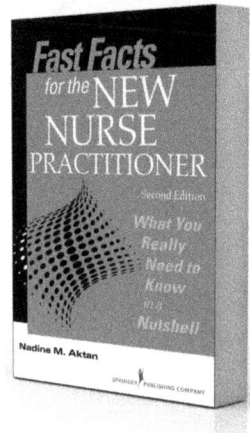
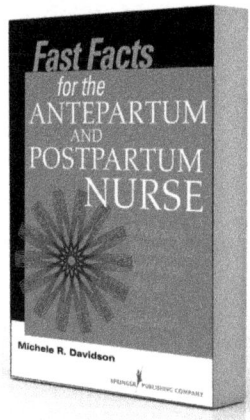
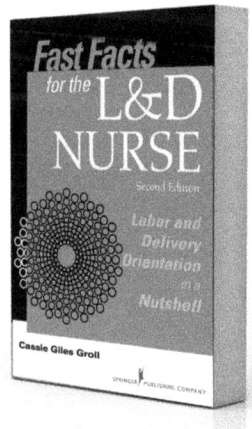
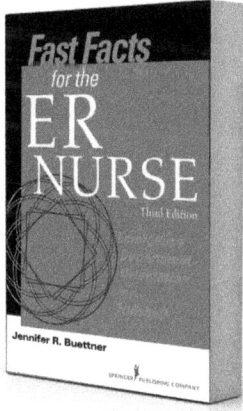

These must-have reference books are packed with timely, useful, and accessible information presented in a clear, precise format. Pocket-sized and affordable, the series provides quick access to information you need to know and use daily.

springerpub.com/FastFacts